T0234533

OTHER FAST FACTS BOOKS

Fast Facts About PTSD: A Guide for Nurses and Other Health Care Professionals (*Adams*)

Fast Facts for the NEW NURSE PRACTITIONER: What You Really Need to Know in a Nutshell, Second Edition (*Aktan*)

Fast Facts for the ER NURSE: Emergency Department Orientation in a Nutshell, Third Edition (*Buettner*)

Fast Facts About GI AND LIVER DISEASES FOR NURSES: What APRNs Need to Know in a Nutshell (*Chaney*)

Fast Facts for the MEDICAL–SURGICAL NURSE: Clinical Orientation in a Nutshell (*Ciocco*)

Fast Facts on COMBATING NURSE BULLYING, INCIVILITY, AND WORKPLACE VIOLENCE: What Nurses Need to Know in a Nutshell (*Ciocco*)

Fast Facts for the NURSE PRECEPTOR: Keys to Providing a Successful Preceptorship in a Nutshell (*Ciocco*)

Fast Facts for the OPERATING ROOM NURSE: An Orientation and Care Guide, Second Edition (*Criscitelli*)

Fast Facts for the ANTEPARTUM AND POSTPARTUM NURSE: A Nursing Orientation and Care Guide in a Nutshell (*Davidson*)

Fast Facts for the NEONATAL NURSE: A Nursing Orientation and Care Guide in a Nutshell (*Davidson*)

Fast Facts Workbook for CARDIAC DYSRHYTHMIAS AND 12-LEAD EKGs (*Desmarais*)

Fast Facts About PRESSURE ULCER CARE FOR NURSES: How to Prevent, Detect, and Resolve Them in a Nutshell (*Dziedzic*)

Fast Facts for the GERONTOLOGY NURSE: A Nursing Care Guide in a Nutshell (*Eliopoulos*)

Fast Facts for the LONG-TERM CARE NURSE: What Nursing Home and Assisted Living Nurses Need to Know in a Nutshell (*Eliopoulos*)

Fast Facts for the CLINICAL NURSE MANAGER: Managing a Changing Workplace in a Nutshell, Second Edition (*Fry*)

Fast Facts for EVIDENCE-BASED PRACTICE IN NURSING: Third Edition (*Godshall*)

Fast Facts for Nurses About HOME INFUSION THERAPY: The Expert's Best Practice Guide in a Nutshell (*Gorski*)

Fast Facts About NURSING AND THE LAW: Law for Nurses in a Nutshell (*Grant, Ballard*)

Fast Facts for the L&D NURSE: Labor & Delivery Orientation in a Nutshell, Second Edition (*Groll*)

Fast Facts for the RADIOLOGY NURSE: An Orientation and Nursing Care Guide in a Nutshell (*Grossman*)

Fast Facts on ADOLESCENT HEALTH FOR NURSING AND HEALTH PROFESSIONALS: A Care Guide in a Nutshell (*Herrman*)

Fast Facts for the FAITH COMMUNITY NURSE: Implementing FCN/Parish Nursing in a Nutshell (*Hickman*)

Fast Facts for the CARDIAC SURGERY NURSE: Caring for Cardiac Surgery Patients in a Nutshell, Second Edition (*Hodge*)

Fast Facts About the NURSING PROFESSION: Historical Perspectives in a Nutshell (*Hunt*)

Fast Facts for the CLINICAL NURSING INSTRUCTOR: Clinical Teaching in a Nutshell, Third Edition (*Kan, Stabler-Haas*)

Fast Facts for the WOUND CARE NURSE: Practical Wound Management in a Nutshell (*Kifer*)

Fast Facts About EKGs FOR NURSES: The Rules of Identifying EKGs in a Nutshell (*Landrum*)

Fast Facts for the CRITICAL CARE NURSE: Critical Care Nursing in a Nutshell (*Landrum*)

Fast Facts for the TRAVEL NURSE: Travel Nursing in a Nutshell (*Landrum*)

Fast Facts for the SCHOOL NURSE: What You Need to Know, Third Edition (*Loschiavo*)

Fast Facts for MANAGING PATIENTS WITH A PSYCHIATRIC DISORDER: What RNs, NPs, and New Psych Nurses Need to Know (*Marshall*)

Fast Facts About SUBSTANCE USE DISORDERS: What Every Nurse, APRN, and PA Needs to Know (*Marshall, Spencer*)

Fast Facts About CURRICULUM DEVELOPMENT IN NURSING: How to Develop and Evaluate Educational Programs in a Nutshell, Second Edition (*McCoy, Anema*)

Fast Facts for the CATH LAB NURSE (*McCulloch*)

Fast Facts About NEUROCRITICAL CARE: A Quick Reference for the Advanced Practice Provider (*McLaughlin*)

Fast Facts for DEMENTIA CARE: What Nurses Need to Know in a Nutshell (*Miller*)

Fast Facts for HEALTH PROMOTION IN NURSING: Promoting Wellness in a Nutshell (*Miller*)

Fast Facts for STROKE CARE NURSING: An Expert Care Guide, Second Edition (*Morrison*)

Fast Facts for the MEDICAL OFFICE NURSE: What You Really Need to Know in a Nutshell (*Richmeier*)

Fast Facts for the PEDIATRIC NURSE: An Orientation Guide in a Nutshell (*Rupert, Young*)

Fast Facts About FORENSIC NURSING: What You Need to Know (*Scannell*)

Fast Facts About the GYNECOLOGICAL EXAM: A Professional Guide for NPs, PAs, and Midwives, Second Edition (*Secor, Fantasia*)

Fast Facts for the STUDENT NURSE: Nursing Student Success in a Nutshell (*Stabler-Haas*)

Fast Facts About RELIGION FOR NURSES: Implications for Patient Care (*Taylor*)

Fast Facts for CAREER SUCCESS IN NURSING: Making the Most of Mentoring in a Nutshell (*Vance*)

Fast Facts for the TRIAGE NURSE: An Orientation and Care Guide, Second Edition (*Visser, Montejano*)

Fast Facts for DEVELOPING A NURSING ACADEMIC PORTFOLIO: What You Really Need to Know in a Nutshell (*Wittmann-Price*)

Fast Facts for the HOSPICE NURSE: A Concise Guide to End-of-Life Care (*Wright*)

Fast Facts for the CLASSROOM NURSING INSTRUCTOR: Classroom Teaching in a Nutshell (*Yoder-Wise, Kowalski*)

Forthcoming FAST FACTS Books

Fast Facts About NEUROPATHIC PAIN: What Advanced Practice Nurses and Physician Assistants Need to Know (*Davies*)

Fact Facts in HEALTH INFORMATICS FOR NURSES (*Hardy*)

Fact Facts About NURSE ANESTHESIA (*Hickman*)

Fast Facts for the CARDIAC SURGERY NURSE, Third Edition (*Hodge*)

Fast Facts for the CRITICAL CARE NURSE: Critical Care Nursing, Second Edition (*Landrum*)

Fast Facts to LOVING YOUR RESEARCH PROJECT: A Stress-Free Guide for Novice Researchers in Nursing and Healthcare (*Marshall*)

Fast Facts for DNP ROLE DEVELOPMENT: A Career Navigation Guide (*Menonna-Quinn, Genova*)

Fast Facts for MAKING THE MOST OF YOUR CAREER IN NURSING (*Redulla*)

Fast Facts About SEXUALLY TRANSMITTED INFECTIONS (STIs): A Nurse's Guide to Expert Patient Care (*Scannel*)

Fast facts for the CLINICAL NURSE LEADER (*Wilcox, Deerhake*)

Fast Facts for the HOSPICE NURSE: A Concise Guide to End-of-Life Care, Second Edition (*Wright*)

Visit www.springerpub.com to order.

FAST FACTS for
THE SCHOOL NURSE

Janice Loschiavo, MA, RN, NJ-CSN, is an adjunct instructor at William Paterson University's Graduate Nursing Division and serves as a field supervisor for New Jersey City University. She had 26 years of experience as a school nurse before retiring from that position in 2007. Ms. Loschiavo has received recognitions for excellence both in teaching and as a school nurse, including the New Jersey City University's Distinguished Alumni Award (2014), the Governor's Teacher Recognition Award (2006–2007), the nomination for Disney Teacher of the Year (2002), the New Jersey State School Nurse of the Year (1994–1995), the Bergen County School Nurse of the Year (1994–1995), and the state nomination for National School Nurse of the Year (1994–1995). While working as a school nurse, she was responsible for participating in Child Study Team meetings; maintaining health records; conducting health screenings; providing first aid to students; teaching health classes; conducting faculty in-service training (anaphylaxis, child abuse, and first aid); organizing health fairs; running workshops for teachers and parents; and serving as liaison to the Division of Youth and Family Services. Ms. Loschiavo contributed to the book *Health Counseling: A Microskills Approach for Counselors, Educators, and School Nurses*, Second Edition, edited by Richard Blonna. ADVANCE for Nurses published her article, "Considering School Nursing?," in January 2013. In 2016, Ms. Loschiavo wrote and published *Life's Lessons for Children*, which provides character education lesson plans for students K to 12.

FAST FACTS for
THE SCHOOL NURSE

What You Need to Know

Third Edition

Janice Loschiavo, MA, RN, NJ-CSN

SPRINGER PUBLISHING COMPANY

Copyright © 2020 Springer Publishing Company, LLC

All rights reserved.

No part of this publication may be reproduced, stored in a retrieval system, or transmitted in any form or by any means, electronic, mechanical, photocopying, recording, or otherwise, without the prior permission of Springer Publishing Company, LLC, or authorization through payment of the appropriate fees to the Copyright Clearance Center, Inc., 222 Rosewood Drive, Danvers, MA 01923, 978-750-8400, fax 978-646-8600, info@copyright.com or on the Web at www.copyright.com.

Springer Publishing Company, LLC
11 West 42nd Street
New York, NY 10036
www.springerpub.com
http://connect.springerpub.com

Acquisitions Editor: Adrianne Brigido
Compositor: Amnet Systems

ISBN: 978-0-8261-7414-7
ebook ISBN: 978-0-8261-7415-4
DOI: 10.1891/9780826174154

19 20 21 22 / 5 4 3 2 1

The author and the publisher of this Work have made every effort to use sources believed to be reliable to provide information that is accurate and compatible with the standards generally accepted at the time of publication. The author and publisher shall not be liable for any special, consequential, or exemplary damages resulting, in whole or in part, from the readers' use of, or reliance on, the information contained in this book. The publisher has no responsibility for the persistence or accuracy of URLs for external or third-party Internet websites referred to in this publication and does not guarantee that any content on such websites is, or will remain, accurate or appropriate.

Library of Congress Cataloging-in-Publication Data

Names: Loschiavo, Janice, author.
Title: Fast facts for the school nurse : what you need to know / Janice Loschiavo.
Description: Third edition. | New York, NY : Springer Publishing Company, LLC, [2020] | Series: Fast facts | Includes bibliographical references and index.
Identifiers: LCCN 2019015850 (print) | LCCN 2019016619 (ebook) | ISBN 9780826174154 (eBook) | ISBN 9780826174147 (print : alk. paper)
Subjects: | MESH: School Nursing—methods | Practice Patterns, Nurses' | Nurses Instruction
Classification: LCC RJ247 (ebook) | LCC RJ247 (print) | NLM WY 113 | DDC 371.7/12—dc23
LC record available at https://lccn.loc.gov/2019015850

Contact us to receive discount rates on bulk purchases.
We can also customize our books to meet your needs.
For more information please contact: sales@springerpub.com

Publisher's Note: New and used products purchased from third-party sellers are not guaranteed for quality, authenticity, or access to any included digital components.

Printed in the United States of America.

This book is dedicated to all
school nurses—past, present, and future.
May we always remember this:
Children cannot interrupt your work.
They are your work.

Contents

Part IV THE MARGINALIZED CHILD

Part V PROBLEMS UNIQUE TO THE SCHOOL NURSE SETTING

Foreword

School nursing is noble work and a recognized specialty within the profession of nursing. Its origin can be traced to the dawn of the 19th century, with Lillian Wald and her founding of the Henry Street Settlement in New York City. Wald and her nurses were politically astute and tenacious in advocating for the health of the community. Their legacy was the establishment of school nursing as a vital part of the community.

School nurses strive to deliver to educators students who are in optimum condition for learning. The mission of the educational system is doomed to failure without the knowledge and skills of school nurses who intervene to solve actual health problems, manage chronic diseases, and promote health and healthful lifestyles. All of this is accomplished within the orientation of the community and the primary system for care for most children—the family.

Of course, success is impossible unless the behaviors of healthful living are instilled in the students themselves. The ultimate goal of school nursing is self-care and personal understanding of the meaning of health and wellness. It starts with having students appreciate the health legacy of the family and how investing in a healthful lifestyle will serve them well throughout life—and further understand, how once lost, health may be difficult to recapture. School nurses convey such understanding through role modeling and the education process. First and foremost, a school nurse is a teacher.

The work of a school nurse is not for the faint of heart, especially in today's milieu of social diversity, complex medical treatments, and expectation that, whenever possible, children with special needs will be mainstreamed to promote lives as close to being normal as possible. For most school nurses, every day is a cacophony of special needs, each to be resolved, each unique and different from every other in its cause and solution. Modern times have brought more attention to student needs: autism spectrum disorders, childhood obesity, drug use (both prescribed and illegal), problems of sexuality and mental health, school violence, child abuse, and cultural diversity, to name a few. It is clear that these issues have to be approached within a team context, but each is inextricably associated with health and demands the holistic perspective that characterizes nursing.

Beyond the human problems that dominate the work of school nursing, there are the legal, ethical, and institutional policies that represent both assistance and obstacles to bringing the best of nursing science to students. *Fast Facts for the School Nurse* is a virtual compendium of situations that school nurses encounter in their practice. It will direct school nurses to the answers for many questions and to wiser counsel when a dilemma seems unsolvable. It is a reference for school nurses authored by a school nurse of publicly acclaimed distinction who brings a lifetime of experience to these pages.

Lucille A. Joel, EdD, RN, FAAN
Distinguished Professor, School of Nursing
Rutgers, The State University of New Jersey
New Brunswick/Newark, New Jersey

Preface

If you are a school nurse, you likely have been asked the same condescending question from nursing colleagues that I have: "How could you have gone from being a fabulous emergency department or intensive care nurse to being a *school nurse*? All you do now is put on Band-Aids and give out tooth-fairy necklaces."

If you do not have a good answer, I will give you mine: "As a school nurse and health teacher, my challenge will be to *prevent* a disease, accident, or illness from occurring in the first place. If I do my job well, there will be far fewer patients in emergency departments and intensive care units."

BACKGROUND

Today's schools are very different from those of the past. They must be, because today's students are also quite different. Children today face challenges unique to the times. They may come from the growing number of unstable homes. Highly addictive, illegal drugs are now easily available. Sexually transmitted infections have always been a concern, but AIDS can carry a death sentence. Other risk factors such as obesity and sedentary lifestyles not only are unhealthful but can also lead to childhood unhappiness. Cultural diversity and environmental issues contribute to feelings of fear and isolation. Mainstreamed children with special needs are particularly vulnerable and in need of much support. Sadly, today's students know fear. Schools can be targets for deranged killers. All of these factors and many more can interfere with a student's ability to learn.

The schools and the people within them often provide the only stability in some children's lives. Therefore, it makes sense that school personnel be educated to recognize the turmoil in such children's lives and offer needed guidance.

It is no secret that an ill, unhappy child simply cannot learn. This book will help school nurses recognize a wide range of health issues and the ever-expanding role that they have in prevention and treatment. In doing so, the school nurse will free children to learn and grow in a safe, nurturing academic environment.

THE PURPOSE OF THIS BOOK

The reader will find this book useful for two purposes. First, it is a quick-reference guide for both the novice and the experienced school nurse who wishes to keep abreast of new information. Part IV, The Marginalized Child, will be particularly helpful in preventing and dealing with some of today's most prevalent health issues.

This book can also serve as a supplemental textbook for nurses who are enrolled in college or university programs of study for state certification or who are preparing to take the examination for national certification through the National Board for the Certification of School Nurses. This book includes relevant information about the five components included in the exam and in the courses that must be taken: health problems and nursing management, health appraisal, health promotion and disease prevention, professional issues, and special health issues.

ORGANIZATION OF THIS BOOK

Part I, School Nursing: Making the Change and Excelling, covers basic elements of the specialty of school nursing. Part II, Health Appraisal in School Nursing: Health Promotion and Disease Prevention, addresses school nurses' role in student assessment and health counseling. Part III, Professional Issues in School Nursing Practice, discusses professional responsibilities of school nurses. Part IV, The Marginalized Child, examines some of the most important health issues that affect students today and what school nurses in their role of nurse and health teacher can do to prevent, recognize early, and manage these issues in the school setting. Part V, Problems Unique to the School Nurse Setting, addresses issues relevant only to school nursing.

NEW FEATURES OF THIS THIRD EDITION

When I began the challenge of writing this new edition, I had no idea of the large number of changes that had taken place in just a few years. I am most excited about several new features included in this edition.

I have added a chapter titled "Up Your Game." This chapter includes descriptions of 12 attributes essential for school nurse practice and simple-to-do assignments so you can *up your game*.

Also included is a separate section dealing with the *marginalized child*. This includes the child struggling with gender identity, mental illness, and chronic health conditions.

Gun violence, the history of drug use in the United States, medical use of marijuana, vaping, and Narcan use are also explored in this new edition.

THE AUTHOR'S GOALS

My goals in writing this book are simple. I wish to share my passion for school nursing and to help my colleagues recognize that their school nursing careers are unique opportunities for helping students and the larger community.

I wish you well and hope that you will find this book not only an essential guide but also a comfort as you meet the exciting professional challenges of school nursing.

Janice Loschiavo

ACKNOWLEDGMENTS

I would like to thank Adrianne Brigido, Director of Nurse Education at Springer Publishing Company, for helping me put together this third edition. She clearly has an understanding of the profession of nursing and appreciation for school nurses. Adrianne "held my hand" to help me make this new edition even better.

Of course, I am ever grateful to my friend, Lucille Joel, for her faith in me and encouragement to reach further to do more and better throughout my career. She continues to serve as my role model, not only as a nurse but as a wife, mother, and grandmother.

I thank my many school nurse colleagues, especially my students who continue to impress me with their knowledge and perseverance and, in doing so, have kept me humble.

I thank Jan Halder for her technological support and dear friendship. I thank the ladies in my writing group—Paula Mate, Jane Paterson, and Tina Segali—for their support and guidance.

I thank my children, Lori, Jill, and Rick, for their understanding when they so often had to share their mother. I thank them also for the gift of grandchildren: Ryan, Ashley, Richard, Luke, Preston, and Austin. These bright, beautiful babies keep me focused on what truly matters in life.

Most of all, I thank my husband, Rich. Rich has learned to tolerate piles of papers and often a most distracted, preoccupied wife. After almost 52 years of marriage, he continues to "hold my hand" and heart as well.

I

School Nursing: Making the Change and Excelling

1

Bed Baths to Band-Aids: What the School Nurse *Really* Does

You might have a number of reasons for wanting a career as a school nurse. Maybe you feel that you are no longer physically or emotionally up to the demands of hospital work. Perhaps you want shorter workdays and work years so that you can spend more time at home, or you are simply tired of being away from your family on weekends and holidays. These certainly are valid reasons for wanting a change.

There may be other, more subtle reasons why you are considering a career as a school nurse. You may be frustrated by caring for patients who are ill because of poor lifestyle choices, interested in helping prevent diseases and accidents, ready to work independently, or seeking a greater professional challenge. If these issues resonate with you, I invite you to join me in the role of school nurse/teacher of health. Together with our colleagues, we can elevate the quality of healthcare for each child. In doing so, we also can raise the level of wellness for schools, communities, and the nation itself.

In this chapter, you will learn:

1. The definition of *school nursing*
2. The history of school nursing and how it is rooted in public health
3. The components of a coordinated school health program
4. Framework for 21st century school nursing practice

5. The importance of the *Healthy People* initiatives
6. The three levels of prevention

DEFINITION

The National Association of School Nurses (NASN, 2017) defines *school nursing* as

> a specialized practice of nursing, protects and promotes student health, facilitates optimal development, and advances academic success. School nurses, grounded in ethical and evidence-based practice, are the leaders who bridge health care and education, provide care coordination, advocate for quality student-centered care, and collaborate to design systems that allow individuals and communities to develop their full potential.

Simply put, school nurses support student achievement through wellness. We are nurses *and* teachers who work to prevent and control illnesses so that students can learn to their greatest potential.

HISTORY

Early Beginnings

Before the 19th century, the United States had little in the way of a formal healthcare delivery system. Births, injuries, illnesses, and deaths were dealt with at home, and caring for family members was an accepted part of everyday life. In the late 1800s, thousands of people immigrated to New York from rural areas of the United States and from Europe. These people were often poor, homeless, hungry, very sick, and far from relatives and friends. With only a fragment of a healthcare delivery system in place, there was no one to tend to their many needs. It was also around this time that New York City enacted legislation requiring students to attend school. The prevalence of contagious diseases, already high in the community, increased as students gathered in school settings. The most common contagious diseases of the time—tuberculosis, pediculosis, ringworm, impetigo, and conjunctivitis—were all transmitted in crowded and unsanitary conditions.

Although compulsory school attendance was a huge step forward in education, it was a recipe for disaster because of the health concerns. It was not unusual for a child to be repeatedly exposed, infected, and excluded from school for the same disease. A child could be permanently truant because of a small curable lesion. Poor children often left school by the age of 14 to take their place in the workforce or to watch their younger siblings while their parents earned a living.

The health needs of the populace were so overwhelming that they presented a tremendous threat to the growth of the city. One woman chose to do something about it. Lillian Wald was a bright young lady from an affluent family who had graduated from the New York Hospital School of Nursing. One day, while she was teaching a class to immigrant women, a young girl asked her to help her very ill mother. Wald made a house call and was appalled by the living conditions of the poor people whom she encountered. She found large families living in single rooms shared with boarders. All the tenants in the building used one toilet, which had no door and seldom worked. Wald was ashamed to be part of a society that allowed conditions like this to exist, and she committed herself to improving the lives of these poor people.

Wald, along with friend and colleague Mary Brewster, founded the Visiting Nurse Service of New York in 1893 with funding from philanthropists and friends. By January of 1894, the two had visited more than 125 families. One year later, Wald moved herself and seven other nurses to 265 Henry Street, a tenement in one of the poorest neighborhoods of New York City. There, she founded the renowned Henry Street Settlement, which still exists today.

The Henry Street Settlement

The Henry Street Settlement was the top floor of the house where the nurses lived and worked. From their home, they were able to easily access those in greatest need, and their patients could reach them. Their patients were referred to as "neighbors."

Wald wanted the Settlement to be a place where all were welcome. She felt strongly that people had to be viewed in totality. Meals were served, the homeless were sheltered, and piano lessons were given to the poor in the dining room. Wald recognized that even the indigent had needs for creative expression. Under her direction, the seeds of many social changes were planted. Wald advocated for child labor laws, park and playground construction, special education, women's suffrage, housing codes, and the profession of school nursing. She was a founding member of the National Association for the Advancement of Colored People (NAACP) and supported funding for "fresh air" programs that would become the Fresh Air Fund.

The Experiment

In 1896, the New York City Department of Health set about addressing the high percentage of absent children in public schools. One hundred fifty of the finest physicians were hired to spend 1 hour a day inspecting schoolchildren. Their focus was to exclude sick children from school. There was no follow-up or teaching of positive health habits. Once children were excluded, they simply did not return to school—ever. Meanwhile, in just a few years, the Henry Street Settlement had grown. Wald was not only a visionary nurse but also a savvy politician. Once she became aware of the failure of the physicians' work, she made an offer to the chancellor of New York City's schools. Wald proposed to provide a nurse who would work in four of the schools with the greatest number of absent and medically excluded children. If the absentee rate significantly decreased, the city would then pay to have a school nurse in every school.

On October 1, 1902, Lina Rogers, one of the eight nurses from the Henry Street Settlement, started her job. She spent 1 hour a day at each school, with a total enrollment of 8,671 students. With limited space and almost no supplies, she dressed wounds, treated conjunctivitis, cleaned skin infections, and excluded children from school when necessary. However, this time, the excluded children received follow-up visits in their homes, where parents were educated about health issues. Rogers recognized the needs of both patient and family; she made referrals, and follow-up care was provided. Children recovered, returned to school, and were able to learn. The program was so successful that 25 more nurses were soon hired. Within 1 year, absenteeism decreased by 90%, and New York City became the first municipality in the world to take financial responsibility for children's health while they were in school. One humble young nurse working in deplorable conditions had succeeded where 150 prominent physicians had failed. Why? She recognized the complexity of the health needs of individuals and offered herself as a nurse, teacher, and friend.

Fast Facts

School nursing has its roots in public health. Nursing pioneers recognized that caring for children in the school setting was an excellent means of controlling disease and that children needed to be well enough to attend school so education could take place. Working conditions were initially deplorable but improved once the school nurses' work became recognized and respected.

(*continued*)

(continued)

Clinical Snapshot

Catherine was thrilled to be hired as a school nurse immediately after graduation. She was not so thrilled when she saw her tiny, hot, inaccessible office with no bathroom nearby. After the initial shock, Catherine rolled up her sleeves and began to work within the system to improve the health office atmosphere and establish herself as an important presence.

As you plan your school nurse practice, remember our public health roots, and accept that although you may have less than perfect working conditions, you can still be an effective school nurse and a dynamic health teacher.

Years of Growth

In the years that followed the New York City experiment, the role of school nurses expanded in concert with the needs of the students and the community. Children were still evaluated and excluded from school when warranted, but the responsibility for health began to shift to the home. School nurses enabled this transition through education. Health education began to emerge as a separate discipline, and certified school nurses were the major force in making the necessary changes.

As World War II loomed, the focus was on national security. Healthy men were needed to serve quickly. Unfortunately, one fourth of all draftees were rejected because of the residual effects of preventable childhood illnesses or malnutrition. It became clear that there were lingering aftereffects of childhood illnesses that, in many instances, could have been avoided with preventive education, early detection, and prompt treatment.

Recognizing these health issues, school nurses began to develop programs and work with teachers to incorporate them into the curriculum. Classes in nutrition were taught to students and parents. Screenings were done, and children with vision or hearing problems were referred and treated. School health services expanded into a comprehensive program, with the school nurse assuming more of a teaching role (Table 1.1).

COMPONENTS OF A COORDINATED SCHOOL HEALTH PROGRAM

The eight-component model of a school health program was originally proposed by Allensworth and Kolbe (1987). Their expanded perspective encouraged links within the school community and

Table 1.1

Historical Timeline of School Nursing

1892	London Amy Hughes is hired to investigate the nutritional status of schoolchildren in the school setting. This is the first recorded employment of a school nurse.
1893	Belgium Brussels is the first city to employ a school physician and establish organized, citywide inspection of schools.
1894	Boston School health services are initiated to identify and exclude students with serious communicable diseases such as pertussis, measles, mumps, scarlet fever, and parasitic diseases, including pediculosis, ringworm, and scabies.
1902	New York The Henry Street Settlement is organized, modeled after an English program. Lillian Wald, head nurse, appoints Lina Rogers as the nation's first school nurse. The goal is to decrease absenteeism following implementation of mandatory school attendance. Between 1902 and 1903, the number of absentees decreases from 10,567 to 1,101. Twenty-five more nurses are then hired and paid by the New York City Board of Education.
1920s	This decade sees the expansion of the school nurse's role. Health education is added, and medical examinations begin in schools to identify physical defects.
1930s	Individual states begin to require specific education for school nurse practice.
1940s	War is present in much of the world. Leaders in the United States realize the importance of the maximum degree of health for all to serve in the armed forces and support the country at home. Health as a school subject begins to include an emphasis on physical fitness. Educators recognize the correlation between health teaching and practice.
1950s	The role of the school nurse is expanded to focus on prevention. Screenings in dental health, vision, and hearing are followed up, and fewer students are left with chronic diseases. Health counseling is introduced.
1960	Some states require nurses to have teaching degrees.
1965	Federal laws begin to take shape ensuring that all children, handicapped or not, are appropriately educated. These laws further strengthen the position of the school nurse, whose presence now is required to perform treatments and give medications in the school setting. These laws continue to be revised, renamed, and enhanced to further benefit all children with special needs.

(continued)

Table 1.1

Historical Timeline of School Nursing (*continued*)

1968	The National Education Association (NEA) establishes the Department of School Nurses (DSN). A nationwide survey is conducted to establish school nurse credentials for each state. The DSN begins to form committees, develop policies, and elect officers.
1979	The DSN separates from NEA to form the National Association of School Nurses (NASN), which now serves as the hub for all the state organizations.
Today	School nursing continues to flourish as a separate discipline. Through NASN, school nurses partner with national health organizations, publish a journal and reference books, formulate position statements, and hold nationwide conventions to disseminate information and foster communication. NASN also employs a Washington, DC–based representative to lobby for school nursing issues and interact with Congress on the organization's behalf.

suggested that time and resources could be better utilized if school health programs were coordinated and comprehensive. A coordinated school health program is intended to serve as an interactive framework across school settings. The eight components are:

1. Health education
2. Physical education
3. Health services
4. Nutrition services
5. Mental health and social services
6. Healthful and safe school environment
7. Health promotion for staff
8. Parent/family and community involvement

FRAMEWORK FOR 21ST CENTURY SCHOOL NURSING PRACTICE

On January 6, 2016, the NASN developed the Framework for 21st Century School Nursing Practice, which better reflects today's school nurse practice. The framework focuses on student-centered nursing care that occurs within the family and the school community.

The key principles include:

1. *Standards of Practice*
   Clinical Competence, Clinical Guidelines, Code of Ethics, Critical Thinking, Evidence-Based Practice, NASN Position Statements, Nurse Practice Acts, Scope and Standards of Practice

2. *Care Coordination*
   Case Management, Chronic Disease Management, Collaborative Communication, Direct Care, Education, Interdisciplinary Teams, Motivational Interviewing/Counseling, Nursing Delegation, Student Care Plans, Student-Centered Care, Student Self-Empowerment, Transition Planning
3. *Leadership*
   Advocacy, Change Agents, Education Reform, Funding and Reimbursement, Healthcare Reform, Lifelong Learner, Models of Practice, Technology, Policy Development and Implementation, Professionalism, Systems-Level Leadership
4. *Quality Improvement*
   Continuous Quality Improvement, Documentation/Data Collection, Evaluation, Meaningful Health/Academic Outcomes, Performance Appraisal, Research, Uniform Data Set
5. *Community/Public Health*
   Access to Care, Cultural Competency, Disease Prevention, Environmental Health, Health Education, Health Equity, *Healthy People 2020*, Health Promotion, Outreach, Population-Based Care, Risk Reduction, Screenings/Referral/Follow-Up, Social Determinants of Health, Surveillance (NASN, 2018)

The ultimate goal of the framework is to provide a unified resource to guide school nurses in their practice by helping students to be healthy, safe, and ready to learn.

HEALTHY PEOPLE INITIATIVES

It has long been recognized that the health of each individual is linked to the health of the community and the health of the community is the foundation for the health of the nation.

In 1979, *Healthy People* was initiated by the U.S. Department of Health and Human Services. It is a comprehensive, nationwide health promotion and disease prevention agenda. It represents a set of national 10-year goals and objectives developed to improve the health of all Americans. These objectives were written after referencing over 8,000 comments from diverse individuals and organizations. *Healthy People* now guides the country by providing a list of priorities for each ensuing decade. At the completion of each decade, the objectives are evaluated and new ones developed to meet the needs of the changing world. In 1990, 226 health objectives were listed. Today, the *Healthy People 2020* initiative encompasses over 1,200 areas to improve our nation's health.

Healthy People is grounded in the principle that setting objectives and monitoring progress can motivate action and behavior change. *Healthy People 2010* saw 23% of its objectives met or exceeded and 48% moved toward the target goal. Thus far, it is estimated that the country has made progress toward or met 71% of its *Healthy People* targets (U.S. Department of Health and Human Services, 2010). See Appendix A for all *Health People 2020* initiatives.

Today's school nurse must be cognizant of ever-changing world needs and respectful of the data presented. With this information we can develop timely health programs for our schools and influence policy making in the communities we live and work within.

Healthy People 2020 Objective:
Educational and Community-Based Programs, 5.1: Increase the proportion of elementary, middle, and high schools that have a full-time, registered, school nurse-to-student ratio of at least 1:750 from 40.6% in 2006 to 44.7%.

HEALTHY PEOPLE 2030

Healthy People 2030 is the fifth edition of *Healthy People.* It aims at new challenges and builds on lessons learned from the first four decades. In June 2018, the Department of Health and Human Services reviewed the proposed framework submitted by the Advisory Committee on National Health Promotion and Disease Prevention, and final approval was received. The framework is to:

- Provide context and rationale for the initiative's approach
- Communicate the principles that underlie decisions about *Healthy People 2030*
- Situate the initiative in the five-decade history of *Healthy People*

Since the *Healthy People* initiative was first launched, the United States has made significant progress. Achievements include reducing major causes of death such as heart disease and cancer; reducing infant and maternal mortality; reducing risk factors like tobacco smoking, hypertension, and elevated cholesterol; and increasing childhood vaccinations. During these decades, the importance of collaborating across agencies at the national, state, local, and tribal levels and with the private and public health sectors has been demonstrated.

Although much progress has been made, the United States still lags other developed countries (such as other members of the Organization for Economic Co-operation and Development [OECD]) on key measures of health and well-being, including life expectancy, infant mortality, and obesity, despite spending the highest percentage of its gross domestic product on health. A challenge for *Healthy People 2030* is to guide the United States in achieving our population's full potential for health and well-being so that we are second to none among developed countries.

LEVELS OF PREVENTION

School nurses differ from hospital nurses in that we deal with prevention, as opposed to intervention. We seek to prevent health problems through education. In the hospital we intervene because a problem already exists and must be fixed. There are three levels of prevention to be considered in the delivery of healthcare in school settings: primary, secondary, and tertiary (Wold, 1981).

Primary Prevention

Primary prevention takes place before an illness or injury occurs. Its measures include health education, basic hygiene, immunizations, and healthful lifestyle practices. This level of prevention is the most cost-effective and efficient.

Secondary Prevention

Once a person is affected by disease, an accident has occurred, or a health issue becomes apparent, school nurses seek to render a diagnosis and offer prompt, effective treatment. By doing so, we stop the progression and lessen the effects of the problem. Measures include first aid, vision or hearing referrals, and exclusion from school.

Tertiary Prevention

Tertiary prevention is needed for students with existing disabilities for which rehabilitation is expected. The goal is to allow students the maximum school experience in the least restrictive environment while dealing with their disabilities.

Prevention Versus Intervention

Primary and secondary prevention are the keys to cost-effective, comprehensive healthcare. Prevention through education is the focus of the school nurse and the main way in which we differ from our nursing colleagues. Tertiary prevention is costly in terms of time, money, and pain.

References

Allensworth, D. D., & Kolbe, L. J. (1987). The comprehensive school health program: Exploring an expanded concept. *Journal of School Health, 57*(10), 409–412.

National Association of School Nurses. (2017). *About school nursing—Definition*. Retrieved from https://www.nasn.org/about-nasn/about

National Association of School Nurses. (2018). *Position Statement. The Role of the 21st Century School Nurse*. Retrieved from https://www.nasn.org/advocacy/professional-practice-documents/position-statements/ps-role

U.S. Department of Health and Human Services. (2010). *Healthy People 2020*. To pics and Objectives. Retrieved from www.healthypeople.gov/2020/topicsobjectives2020/

Wold, S. J. (1981). *School nursing: A framework for practice* (pp. 3–17, 20–29, 39–47). North Branch, MN: Sunrise River Press.

2

Up Your Game: 12 Essential Qualities for Effective School Nurse Practice

Whether you are a rookie or veteran school nurse, there will come a day when you will wonder if you possess what it takes to be an effective school nurse.

A new nurse can quickly become overwhelmed with the prospect of working independently and might even question if he or she made the right career choice. The veteran needs ongoing reassurance he or she is doing a good job and should look for ways and opportunities to do even better.

Today's school nurse is recognized for playing a vital part in the school environment. To fulfill this role, certain qualities are important for any nurse, but for school nurses, these qualities are essential. They represent the pillars of our profession. Once you become adept at demonstrating these attributes, you will be held in the highest esteem by students, parents, and colleagues. The inevitable, human errors you will make will most likely be forgotten and forgiven, since most children, parents, and colleagues will have had many previous interactions with you and know your intent is good.

Recognize that fate frequently places you in situations much larger than you can completely understand. There are times when an issue at hand will leave you feeling insecure and poorly prepared to competently address and remedy it. Be alert to these new challenges and receptive to the influences placed before you. Each event will create a better you—more confident, more capable.

The following pages cover 12 important skills you will need to up your game as a school nurse. Pick one to focus on each month until the behavior becomes instinctive. Keep a personal diary of how and when you applied the specific skill, and reward yourself with a pat on the back. Share your accomplishments with a fellow school nurse. Your colleague will applaud you as well.

In this chapter, you will learn:

1. Twelve essential qualities for effective school nurse practice
2. Tips to help you identify and enhance these personal qualities
3. Realistic assignments to help you learn and grow

1. EMBRACE PROFESSIONAL PRIDE

Professionalism is not about what work you do, it is about how well you do the work.

Amit Kalantri

Do you recognize the value of the school nurse profession?

The profession of school nursing should bring with it a feeling of immense pride and deep pleasure in the opportunity to accomplish wonderful things for children and the school community.

Parents have no choice. They must leave their children daily for at least 6 hours, and for many children, the school day is even longer. While they are apart, parents rely on school personnel to meet their child's physical and emotional needs so learning can take place. The school nurse serves as the bridge between the home and school. Teachers change each year or semester, but the school nurse is a constant presence in that child's school experience.

Here are some suggestions to foster professional pride:

- *Autograph your work with excellence.* Give every task/problem/incident your best effort.
- *Build a reputation for caring.* You accomplish this one student at a time. Answer every email and phone message, even if it is just to say, "I am sorry, but I cannot help you with this issue."

- *Embrace your role.* You are a vital part of the school. No one else can do your job. Recognize your own importance. Understand the bigger picture and your role in making things happen. If undecided about a particular situation, keep the child's best interest in the forefront. Let that guide you.
- *Add to your knowledge base.* Continue to learn by attending workshops, reading journals, and growing your experience.
- *Remember your worth. You are accomplishing what many others could not. Be proud of that.*

Fast Facts

School nursing is quite different from other subspecialties of nursing. Until you actually take on the responsibility of a school health office, you will not fully understand the role.

Clinical Snapshot

School nurse Theresa sometimes wonders if she made the right career choice. She finds that working without colleagues can be lonely and wishes she had another nurse in the office to talk to. Grade levels and departments all have ready-made groups, but Theresa is the only nurse. No one knows what she does or seems to care. Most colleagues feel unless there is a class of 25 students before her, she is not working. Theresa makes half of what a hospital nurse makes and has twice the responsibility. She knew all this before, but now living it is painful.

Remedy:

Recall the days when she was upset in her previous job and why she chose school nursing.

Reach out to school nurse colleagues in the district, county, or state for support.

To-Do Assignment:

Keep a daily diary of good things you did that day: the child you consoled, the hearing defect you identified, a lesson that went well, a compliment you received. Write and read before you leave for the day. Remind yourself of these deeds instead of dwelling on things you wish you had done better.

2. HONE YOUR COMMUNICATION SKILLS

The most important thing in communication is hearing what isn't said.

Peter Drucker

Do you speak and write well?

Communication is much more than words going from one person's mouth to another's ears. We communicate in a variety of ways. In addition to words, messages are transmitted by the tone and quality of your voice, eye contact, physical closeness, and overall body language.

Verbal communication must be clear. It requires straightforward language that is direct and honest and sensitive to the situation. *Nonverbal* can be much more difficult to interpret. It consists of your body language and cues that you give off while listening.

Effective communication must include good eye contact. Eye contact is a communication connector and confirms attention and interest between individuals. When you smile and relax, you will appear more approachable.

Keep in mind that today written communication is often overlooked in favor of electronic shorthand or other nonverbal, quicker means. When the question or response required is detailed, only a conversation will do. Too often, emails or texted information is misunderstood.

The school nurse is frequently called upon to write reports, memos, or letters. How well one writes is a direct reflection on that person. Spelling errors and poor wording confuse the reader and detract from the message.

Fast Facts

Most school nurses work independently in the health office with no assistance. Completing required tasks without interruptions can be very difficult.

Clinical Snapshot

Theresa resents the frequent interruptions, especially when she is in the middle of writing. She often refuses to even look up when a student/parent enters her office.

Remedy:

If the writing is urgent, explain that to the person, and ask him or her to wait until you are finished.

(*continued*)

(continued)

If possible, put off writing tasks until students have left your office and the building is less hectic.

Before attending a meeting, make a list of objectives that include the key points you wish to make. Reference these points during the meeting, and make sure they are covered.

To-Do Assignment:

If you struggle with effectively communicating, try modeling yourself after a colleague who does speak and write well. Ask that person to critique you and offer suggestions for improvement.

3. BUILD YOUR LISTENING SKILLS

One of the most sincere forms of respect is actually listening to what another has to say.

Bryant H. McGill

Are you an active listener?

Being a good listener is imperative for school nurses. It is the most fundamental component of interpersonal communication skills. People want and need to be listened to, not just heard. Active, attentive listening is a skill that you can easily acquire and develop with practice.

Active listening is simply paying attention to the speaker. All senses are involved. It involves concentrating, engaging, and absorbing what the person is saying. You must display obvious body language messages such as making good eye contact, smiling, mirroring facial expressions, and reinforcing responses such as nodding and asking for clarification as necessary. This will demonstrate that you understand, and it opens an opportunity for correction if you have misunderstood. Summarize the person's key points, and then state clearly what you can and cannot do to help him or her. Avoid distractions such as fidgeting, checking the clock or your watch, and so on.

The benefits of active listening are obvious.

- Students and staff will trust and respect your interest.
- The speaker will feel valued and understood (Seek, n.d.).

- You will be better able to diffuse conflict. By being open to the entire issue, resolution can be achieved equitably.
- If you listen carefully and understand the issues that are causing your students stress, you will understand them and the staff better. Empathy will easily come to you.
- You will see the problem in different light and be able to help with the solution.

Fast Facts

Listening attentively is hard for Theresa. She simply does not know how to handle distractions and stay focused.

Clinical Snapshot

Establish a routine for yourself. When someone enters your office to speak with you, put down your pen, turn away from the computer, establish eye contact, and smile and adopt a listening pose.

Remedy:

Practice active listening skills. If possible, come from behind the desk, and sit at a table across from the speaker. Nod frequently, maintain good eye contact, and ask for clarification as needed.

To-Do Assignment:

After someone has spoken with you, review the preceding suggestions: eye contact, mirroring, clarification, and so on. Rate yourself, and seek to improve each interaction.

4. CULTIVATE CURIOSITY

Curiosity is one of the greatest secrets of happiness.

Bryant H. McGill

Do you have an active mind?

School nursing can be boring! If you limit your day to rendering first aid, doing screenings, checking immunizations, and completing necessary reports, boredom and monotony will define your role.

Curiosity is a state of active interest or genuinely wanting to know more about something. It allows you to embrace unfamiliar circumstances, giving you a greater opportunity to experience discovery and joy. Curiosity and seeking new information drives achievement, and the degree of curiosity can relate to your personal growth opportunities and how effectively you connect with people.

Curiosity is perhaps the most important attitude. Life is better and more rewarding when you are curious. Simply put, curiosity is the desire to learn, understand, and grow. As we are part of a profession that continues to evolve, having curiosity will lead to enthusiasm and willingness to seek new challenges.

Do not let fear hinder your curiosity. Ask the hard questions. Curiosity is making the choice to look deeper into everyday things to see their true significance. Realizing there is much to learn from everyone and everything you encounter is the first step to living a fulfilling and happy life.

Much like muscles in our body, the mind needs to be exercised and opened for new ideas and challenges. There is no better mental exercise than curiosity. Without a healthy curiosity, opportunities for growth will pass you by and be lost.

It is vital that you adopt an attitude of inquisitiveness and remain open minded about learning new things. Do not hesitate to challenge the status quo. Indifference and malaise is a death sentence. Be willing to try a new approach to a problem. Take the risk, and do not fear failure.

Yes, school nursing, like any other profession, can be repetitive and boring. It is up to you to make it not so. Continue to learn, grow, and ask questions. Do not become complacent in your work. Curiosity is a wonderful tool to have.

Fast Facts

Be alert for harmful, insidious health issues that could develop in students or staff.

Clinical Snapshot

Theresa was curious why a disproportionate number of students in one wing of the building were coming to her with complaints of headaches. She walked over to the classrooms in the wing and noted an unpleasant odor. At her suggestion, air quality studies were done, revealing a slow gas leak previously undetected.

Remedy:

Ask yourself why a situation is happening. Rather than just putting on the bandage or handing over the aspirin, investigate why

(*continued*)

(continued)

children are falling on the playground. Is the equipment safe? Is supervision adequate? Is the environment hazard free? Prevention will save time and pain in the long run.

To-Do Assignment:

Learn one new thing every day. It could be a new computer skill, new school policy, or new student's name and background.

5. MAINTAIN A SENSE OF HUMOR

The most wasted of days is a day without laughter.

Charlie Chaplin

Can you find humor in daily events?

Much of what we do is no cause for merriment. It is sad, serious, and overwhelming. Therefore, it is essential that you look for opportunities to laugh and enjoy your role. Remember that there is also great joy in what you give to others around you.

Do not take every issue seriously. Sure, what we do is serious business, but many experts say if you are not laughing, you are not learning. It matters not what happens in our day but how we react to the issue. Remember that sarcasm is seldom a helpful response.

Laughter has been proven to enhance the health of children by providing a joyful, nonthreatening atmosphere. Adding humor is a great way to communicate and relieves stress. Young children will not be able to define this exactly, but they will appreciate the relief of anxiety.

Fast Facts

A cheerful, positive attitude leads to positive events. Everyone could use more good experiences in his or her day, especially today's student.

Clinical Snapshot

Amy and Christopher, two kindergarten students, entered the health office, holding hands. Amy, serving as the attorney, spoke on behalf of Christopher. "Christopher ate all the fish food." "What?

(continued)

(continued)

Why?" Theresa stammers. Christopher nods in agreement, proud of his accomplishment. Amy adds, "He always eats a little of the fish food, but today he ate the whole box."

Remedy:

Remind Christopher that he should not eat anything without permission from an adult, place the call to poison control for advisement, notify Christopher's parents, and buy more fish food for the teacher.

To-Do Assignment:

Keep a diary of humorous events, and periodically read for your enjoyment. Share with colleagues.

6. DEMONSTRATE FLEXIBILITY

It is not the strongest of the species that survives, it is the one that adapts successfully to change.

Charles Darwin

Are you willing to alter plans and routines?

The need for flexibility in the school setting has never been greater. Your ability to adapt to the ever-changing student, parent, teacher, administrator, and family configurations; gender identity issues; and state and local regulations will mean the difference between growth and stagnation, success and failure.

Far too many school nurses refuse to adopt something new simply because of all the newness surrounding it. We fear that the new request or concept compromises our personal values, is just too difficult, or we resent that our normal routine has been disrupted. We do recognize that progress is important but do not want the associated, inevitable changes it also brings.

To adapt you must be willing to bend and find the *new* right way! The effectively adaptable person meets the other person's needs as well as his or her own.

Fast Facts

It is hard, for some impossible, to set aside personal/religious bias.

(continued)

(*continued*)

Clinical Snapshot

Despite recent state and school policy, Theresa does not believe that transgender youth should be permitted to use the bathroom of the sex they identify with. She makes no secret of her objections and refuses to discuss the issue with administration.

Remedy:

Reevaluate your own bias behavior and seek professional advice. There is no room for discrimination in the health office.

To-Do Assignment:

Consider all the activities and requirements that have changed in recent years. Look closely at the overall picture of education and medicine. Make a list of advantages and disadvantages of these changes. Reconsider your need to be flexible.

7. FOSTER INTERPERSONAL SKILLS

> *People will forget what you say. People will forget what you did—but people will never forget how you made them feel.*
>
> Maya Angelou

Do you have people skills?

Interpersonal skills are a set of abilities that enable us to interact positively and effectively with others. We use them every day when we deal with students, colleagues, and parents. Many associate these skills with emotional intelligence. An emotionally intelligent person can understand what motivates others and how to communicate best with them.

Interpersonal skills are more and more important in today's world of high technology. They are considered the building blocks of communication, much needed when collaboration with others is required (Mindvalley, 2019).

Some of the interpersonal skills most essential for school nurses include collaboration, problem-solving, conflict resolution, empathy, diplomacy, compassion, and patience. We learn these skills as we mature and can hone them as we grow professionally.

Fast Facts

School personnel will inevitably seek your counsel. You will find that it is assumed that you will be fair and nonjudgmental.

Clinical Snapshot

Theresa has become the sounding board as conflicts arise in her school. The principal likes to confide in her about colleagues, students frequently have peer issues, and parents constantly like to complain about teachers.

Remedy:

Listen, and then redirect complainers back to the individual they are having difficulty with, or refer to another school resource if appropriate. Do not side with any one party.

To-Do Assignment:

Be alert for individuals who try to spend too much of your time with complaints.

8. EXHIBIT TRUSTWORTHINESS

> *Trust is like your blood pressure. It is silent, vital to good health and if abused, can be deadly.*
>
> Frank Sonnenberg

Do you have the nine traits of a trustworthy person?

To achieve even moderate success as a school nurse, you must be totally trustworthy. You cannot demand trust any more than you can respect. It must be earned over time. It comes with consistently being honest, acting with integrity, never deliberately being misleading, or lying. It is how you act. It is you. Do you have these traits? (Success, 2015).

1. Are you authentic?
   Authentic people are not arrogant. They are humble, likeable, and easy to talk to.
2. Are you consistent?
   Everyone has said or done something he or she regrets. We all have those days. Children, and occasionally staff, will need your consistent, positive behavior.

3. **Do you have integrity?**
   Do you advocate for what you believe in? Do you support the student or colleague even when others might not?
4. **Are you compassionate?**
   Trustworthy people are compassionate and empathetic. They see themselves in the person's position and think and feel for them.
5. **Are you kind?**
   Do you hold in confidence information that is private? Trustworthy people are kind above all else.
6. **Are you resourceful?**
   Do you constantly seek to learn and grow? As you grow, you support others as well.
7. **Are you a connector?**
   Do you seek to identify with positive people you can learn from?
8. **Are you humble?**
   Do you use your authority to humble people, or are you humble? Are you a good team player?
9. **Are you available?**
   Do you follow up with phone calls after hours? Do you make time for others?
   (Bazin, 2015)

Fast Facts

As much as you want and need to be part of a group, understand that your role is different. You must be available for all and cannot be part of any one group.

Clinical Snapshot

Theresa is frequently invited to have coffee in the teacher's lounge. On the rare occasions that she does join the faculty, she has not been comfortable. Conversations seem to center around students and personal family issues. Theresa will not contribute to gossip and is concerned that she might be seen as part of this negative group.

Remedy:

Remain confident that participating in these discussions is not appropriate. When asked a specific question, explain that you cannot share personal information. If this response is not respected, then do not go into the teacher's lounge.

(continued)

(continued)

To-Do Assignment:

Consider each of the preceding nine characteristics. Check off those you possess, and focus on developing the rest.

9. DEVELOP DECISION-MAKING SKILLS

The road of life is paved with flat squirrels who could not make a decision.

Author Unknown

Do you make the best decision considering the needs of the child first?

Decisions should be made when they are based on sound evidence. Much of what we do as school nurses falls into a gray area. The right decision is not always clear and will depend on your knowledge base, intuition, and past experiences. It is easy to make the decision to call 911 if a child cannot breathe, but most times it is not that clear. You may not like the air exchange you hear, but the child is not gasping for air and assures you all is fine. The child presents with suspicious bruises but denies being hit by his father. Decisions!

Decision-making is the act of choosing between two or more courses of action. Most of us use a combination of intuition, reasoned process, gut instinct, past experiences, and personal values. Reasoning is applying or analyzing the facts before you to make the decision.

Sometimes intuition is fine for the small decisions. Big decisions require a better, structured approach with just a little intuition (SkillsYouNeed, 2018).

You might ask, What is the child's respiratory rate? How is the skin color? Does the child appear anxious? What does the body language tell you? How does this child's lung sounds differ from other children? Does your decision feel right?

Best advice: If in doubt, ship them out! A child's respiratory status can change dramatically in a few seconds.

Make your decision, and commit to it. Do not be swayed by others. Display confidence,and believe in yourself. You are the health professional paid to make the decision (SkillsYouNeed, n.d.).

Fast Facts

Remember your role as part of the team to report suspicion of abuse.

(continued)

(continued)

Clinical Snapshot

A second grader arrives in Theresa's office first thing in the morning. He is bleeding profusely from the nose and has a 1-inch laceration on his upper lip. The student states that his mother hit him. You know the mother well and trust that this was an accident or isolated incident. You call home, and the mother claims that he tripped over his backpack and hit his face on a cabinet. You believe the mother. She is your friend and you trust her.

Two days later, the gym teacher notices the same child has extensive welts on both legs and the child states that his mom hit him with a belt.

You now report this to Child Protective Services, sick that you did not report the first incident and allowed a child to go home to an unsafe environment.

Remedy:

Never let personal relationships interfere with carrying out district policies and procedures.

To-Do Assignment:

When confronted with an important decision, take just a few seconds to weigh the pros and cons of your decision. You must be totally comfortable with your choice of actions.

10. EMBRACE RESPECT

Respect yourself and others will respect you.

Confucius

Do you respect people's right to be different and disagree with you? There are many days you will work under pressure. The office will be filled with ill or injured students, you will have an angry parent on the phone, and you might already be late to teach a class.

Grace under stress will earn you recognition. No matter how you are tested, always retain your diplomacy and poise.

Before you can respect others, you must respect yourself. This simply means that you should see your own worth as a contributing member of the school team. Once you learn to respect yourself, you will find it easier to respect others.

You have absolutely no control over with whom you will work. Every school in this country is diversified. Respect will be the foundation of your success, which will arise from working in a diverse environment. Ethnic differences, racial minorities, gender identity issues, and the learning disabled will thrive only in an atmosphere of mutual respect. Let it begin in your office and classroom.

Respect is one of humankind's most noble sentiments. The highest levels of respect are always earned—never given (Good Choices Good Life, n.d.).

Strive to earn that respect every day, from everyone you deal with: colleagues, parents, and, most of all, children.

Fast Facts

Most likely the health office is located close to the main entrance. Some might perceive you as the official welcoming committee.

Clinical Snapshot

Theresa has a number of parents who like to stop and say hello when they enter the building. She does not mind the quick visit but needs to make it clear that she is there for the students and their needs come first.

Remedy:

Request that a parent visit another time if there are students in the office needing your attention.

To-Do Assignment:

List those individuals in your life whom you honestly respect. Note the reasons you feel this way toward them, and model that behavior.

11. AIM FOR WITH-IT-NESS

The best nurses/teachers do not have special powers but they know how to prevent small stuff from becoming big.

Unknown

With-it-ness is the ability to stay in the moment and remain focused on the task at hand. Remember that *life happens in real time.*

> *Nothing has happened in the past; it happened in the Now. Nothing will ever happen in the future; it will happen in the Now.*
>
> Eckhart Tolle

Can you remain focused and engaged from the moment you enter your office until you leave for the day? Do you put your personal problems in separate compartments to deal with at a later time?

It is a wonderful feeling to be totally involved in what you are doing. That is working in the now. When you recognize that feeling of complete presence, you will incorporate that feeling more and more into your everyday work (Manning, 1988).

Fast Facts

School nurses are responsible to many. Always make the student your priority.

Clinical Snapshot

Many days Theresa does not know where to begin. No matter how early she arrives, there are students waiting for her. She never takes breaks and seldom has an uninterrupted lunch. She stays well after other school personnel leave yet still feels she has accomplished little.

Remedy:

Set aside procedural tasks and care for direct needs of students first.

After the child's needs are met, begin doing the thing you least want to do first. (Make that dreaded phone call, write that report, etc.) Concentrate on one task at a time. Do each task slowly and deliberately and to the best of your ability.

To-Do Assignment:

Formulate a realistic list of what you want to accomplish each day, week, and month. At the end of the day, check your list. Cross off what you have done, and carry over to the next day what you did not get to do. Feel good about your ability to accomplish so much!

12. DISPLAY SELF-CONFIDENCE

Confidence is what you have before you understand the problem.
Woody Allen

Do you believe in yourself? Do you know what your boundaries are? Are you a good role model?

If the answer to these three questions is yes, then you are a confident school nurse. The correct level of self-confidence in yourself and your profession can help you gain the recognition you deserve. It will improve the way people see you, and your decisions will be taken more seriously. Confidence also helps you deal with challenging situations effectively and allows you to seek new goals.

School nurses need to take the initiative and allow themselves to develop confidence in dealing with people. This is especially important when you are dealing with a crisis. Self-confidence will help you remain calm and while accepting the challenges.

Confidence will shape the foundation of your endurance. Your confidence will encourage the parent to allow testing on his or her child, permit the teacher to try a new approach in dealing with a troubled child, or allow the administrator to trust your judgment.

To be successful, it is important to demonstrate self-confidence at every stage of your career, whether you are a new graduate looking for that first position or a more experienced nurse hoping to make a change. Self-confidence at work will improve the way people see you and your views. Ideas and opinions will be taken more seriously. Confidence also enables you to deal with challenging situations more effectively and allows you to set and reach new goals.

Fast Facts

Administrators, faculty, staff, parents, and students need to recognize you as the health professional trained to make assessments.

Clinical Snapshot

Theresa was summoned to the gym where she found a fourth grader lying on the floor, crying in pain, and holding his left shin. The gym teacher claimed that he must have twisted his leg and pulled a muscle. The teacher was attempting to get the student to stand and *walk it off*.

(continued)

(continued)

Theresa thanked the gym teacher and told her, "I will take it from here." Theresa directed someone to call 911 and not to touch the child. She applied ice and splinted the child's leg. Later the child was found to have a fractured fibula.

Remedy:

The gym teacher's intent was good, but Theresa was responsible for the child. Her confident tone and actions established her authority and prevented further injury to the child.

To-Do Assignment:

Speak privately with the gym teacher or any intrusive colleague, and clarify your roles. If you find that you are unsure of your assessment skills, seek to gain more experience. Take any available courses on orthopedic injuries, and consider working a few hours a week in an urgent care center or hospital emergency department.

SUMMARY

The seeds of all the preceding qualities are in each one of us. It only takes a conscious effort to plant them, watch them bud, and continue to blossom as we nurture those around us.

Once you develop these skills, you will be proud, bask in the glow of achievement, and broaden even further what you are capable of accomplishing as school nurses.

Not only will you *up-your-game* as an effective school nurse, but you will find even greater level of self-fulfillment.

References

Bazin, C. (2015). *9 traits of trustworthy people.* Success. Retrieved from https://www.success.com/9-traits-of-trustworthy-people/

Good Choices Good Life. (n.d.). *How to respect yourself and others.* Retrieved from http://www.goodchoicesgoodlife.org/choices-for-young-people/r-e-s-p-e-c-t/

Manning, M. (1988). *Strategies for improving student behavior.* Retrieved from www.greenup.kyschool.us/Downloads/Tips%20for%20Imporving%20Behavior.pdf

Mindvalley. (2019). *What are interpersonal skills and why are they so important?* Retrieved from https://blog.mindvalley.com/what-are-interpersonal-skills/

Seek (n.d.). *3 reasons why active listening is a must-have skill.* Retrieved from https://www.seek.com.au/career-advice/3-reasons-why-active-listening-is-a-must-have-skill

SkillsYouNeed. (2018). *Decision making.* Retrieved from https://www.skillsyouneed.com/ips/decision-making.html

SkillsYouNeed. (n.d.). *Effective Decision-Making.* Retrieved from https://www.skillsyouneed.com/ips/decision-making.html

Success. (2015). *9 traits of trustworthy people.* Retrieved from http://www.success.com/blog/9-traits-of-trustworthy-people

3

Educational Preparation for the School Nurse

Now that you have decided to take on this new professional challenge, you will need to prepare yourself—mentally, physically, and academically. This preparation is important and will not be easy. If it were, many more would choose school nursing.

Begin by exploring your state regulations for school nurse practice. Once you know what must be done, spend some time in a school health office before you invest your money and commit to a career that might be quite different from what you previously perceived.

In this chapter, you will learn:

1. The National Association of School Nurses' (NASN) recommended minimum educational criteria
2. The requirements for national school nurse certification
3. The requirements for educational preparation as a school nurse in your state
4. The scope of practice of the school nurse
5. School nursing subspecialties
6. The future of school nursing

NATIONAL ASSOCIATION OF SCHOOL NURSES' EDUCATIONAL RECOMMENDATIONS

School nurses are part of two disciplines: nursing and education. The NASN in a 2016 position statement established minimum educational criteria for the school nurse:

> It is the position of the National Association of School Nurses (NASN) that every school-age child should have access to a registered professional school nurse (hereinafter referred to as the school nurse), who has a *minimum of* a baccalaureate degree in nursing from an accredited college or university and is licensed as a registered nurse through a board of nursing. These requirements constitute minimal preparation needed to practice at the entry level of school nursing (American Nurses Association [ANA] & NASN, 2011). Additionally, NASN supports state school nurse certification and endorses national certification of school nurses through the National Board for Certification of School Nurses (NBCSN). (NASN, 2016a, 2016b)

Fast Facts

In 1791, the Tenth Amendment to the Constitution was passed, giving the rights of education to the individual states, *not* the federal government. This means that states that are geographically close may have entirely different educational requirements.

Clinical Snapshot

Mary Beth was relieved to learn that she only needed a few credits in addition to her bachelor's degree to become certified as a school nurse in her state. She had never worked in a school but liked the schedule, which would allow her to be home with her children in the afternoons and in summer.

Before jumping into this new challenge, Mary Beth should be certain that she fully understands what a school nurse does. The role of a school nurse might actually be quite different from her perception, and it may not be work she enjoys. It would be prudent if she offered to substitute for a while to be certain this is what she wants to do *before* enrolling in certification courses and spending valuable time and money.

Mary Beth must also look objectively at the change in salary. The workday and work year may be shorter, but the pay will probably be less as well.

Educational Preparation

With few exceptions, school nurses work independently. Their abilities, education, experience, and job performance must be exceptional. It is essential that school nurses know the specific regulations in their state so that they practice within the law.

Fast Facts

As the school nurse's role continues to expand, initiatives and laws are developed that support and guide our practice. These laws are continually changing to meet the needs of our ever-changing society.

Clinical Snapshot

School nurse Mary Beth worked for years at a school in her home district. When her husband was transferred out of state, Mary Beth sought employment in the new school system. She was dismayed to learn that she had to return to school for further coursework to qualify for employment.

All states require some specific preparation to work in a school. Many go beyond this to require a bachelor's degree and certification. Certification is a commitment of value, and the burden is on states to define and demand a minimum but appropriate level of preparation for their school health practitioners (Schwab & Gelfman, 2001, p. 499).

An extensive study of the individual state regulations for school nurse practice was conducted by Praeger and Zimmerman (2009). The following is a summary of their findings:

- All states authorize registered nurses to provide health services; 30 states require state school nurse credentials.
- Thirty-one states have health department staff to provide school nurse coverage.
- Twenty-three states mention licensed practical or vocational nurses as being able to provide school services, but their practice might be limited.
- A baccalaureate degree for the registered nurse is specified in 25 states, with nine of those stipulating that it must be in nursing.
- Twenty-seven states require a school nurse credential, whether it be a license or certificate, to be recognized as a school nurse.

- Twenty-nine states have the department of education authorize the title of school nurse, and 23 receive authorization from the local school districts. Table 3.1 contains an outline of all data contained in this study.

National School Nurse Certification

National school nurse certification is offered through the National Board for Certification of School Nurses (NBCSN). To be eligible to sit for the NBCSN examination, the candidate must meet these requirements:

- Possess a valid license as a registered nurse in one of the states in the United States.
- Have completed a baccalaureate degree in nursing or a health-related field.
- Commencing January 2020, a BSN or higher will be required.
- Have 3 years of experience as a school nurse (NBCSN, 2012).
- The better prepared the school nurse is, the better she will function in the school setting. Even when a degree or specific courses are not required by the state, it is important for the school nurse to continuously seek educational opportunities to enhance her job performance.

Fast Facts

We have all worked with wonderful nurses, but we also know of some nurses who are not so wonderful. A work situation is often manageable because we focus on each other's greater strengths and work as a team. In a school setting, there is no other nurse or team member; thus, it is not enough to be a satisfactory school nurse. Every school nurse must be an outstanding school nurse.

Clinical Snapshot

Mary Beth is finding that the most difficult part of her new school nurse job is the lack of nurse colleagues. The nature of the position separates her from the other teachers and staff. Mary Beth will need to find school nurse role models within the district or county and establish relationships with these nurses. Although they cannot work alongside her, these are the colleagues who will mentor and support her.

Table 3.1

State Regulations for School Nurse (SN) Practice

State	Authorized to Provide Health Services in Schools	Criteria for Becoming a SN	Source of Title	SN Protected Title	SN Mandate	Renewal Requirement
AL	LPN, RN, MD, U	LPN, RN	Dist		X	
AK	RN*, PHN, MD	RN*, Bacc-Ed	DoE	X		Ed
AZ	RN*	RN*	BoN	X		BSN/Ed/CE
AR	LPN, RN, HD, MD, U	RN*	Dist		X	Ed
CA	RN*, MD, D	RN*-Bacc-Ed	DoE	X		Ed, exp
CO	LPN, RN, RN*, HD, MD, D, U	RN*-Bacc-exp-NC	DoE	X		Ed/CE
CT	LPN, RN, RN*, MD, D	RN-exp-Ed/CE	Dist	X	X	CE
DC	LPN, RN, HD, MD, U	LPN, RN	DoH		X	
DE	RN*	RN*-BSN/BaccSchNsg. exp	DoE	X	X	CE/Ed
FL	LPN, RN, HD, MD, D, U	LPN, RN	Dist			
GA	LPN, RN, HD	LPN, RN	Dist		X	
HI	PHN, U	PHN	DoH			
ID	RN*	RN*	DoE	X		Bacc/Ed-exp
IL	RN*, MD	RN*-Bacc-Ed-exp	DoE	X	X	CE
IN	LPN, RN*	RN*-BSN	DoE	X	X	Ed
IA	RN, RN*	RN, RN*-Bacc, RN*-BSN-exp	Dist, DoE	X	X	Ed

(continued)

Table 3.1

State Regulations for School Nurse (SN) Practice (*continued*)

State	Authorized to Provide Health Services in Schools	Criteria for Becoming a SN	Source of Title	SN Protected Title	SN Mandate	Renewal Requirement
KS	LPN, RN*	RN*-BSN	DoE	X	X	Ed
KY	LPN, RN, RN*, MD	RN*-exp, RN*-Bacc-exp/NC	DoE	X		Ed/CE, exp
LA	RN*, U	RN*-exp, RN*-Bacc-exp	DoE	X	X	Ed, exp
ME	RN*, MD	RN*-Bacc-exp	DoE	X	X	Ed/CE
MD	RN, HD, MD, U	RN-Ed	Dist, DoH			CE
MA	RN*, MD	RN*-BSN-Ed/NC	DoE	X	X	Ed, NC
MI	RN*, HD, U	RN*-exp-Ed/Bacc	DoE	X		Ed
MN	RN*, PHN	RN*-BSN-PHN	DoE	X	X	CE
MS	LPN, RN, HD, MD	RN	Dist		X	
MO	LPN, RN, HD, MD	RN	Dist		X	
MT	LPN, RN, HD, MD, D, U	LPN, RN	Dist			
NE	LPN, RN, RN*, HD, MD, D, U	RN*-Ed	DoE	X		Ed
NY	RN*, HD, U	RN*Bacc-Ed/NC, RN*-BSN	DoE	X		
NH	LPN, RN, HD, MD, D, U	RN	Dist	X	X	

(continued)

Table 3.1

State Regulations for School Nurse (SN) Practice (*continued*)

State	Authorized to Provide Health Services in Schools	Criteria for Becoming a SN	Source of Title	SN Protected Title	SN Mandate	Renewal Requirement
NJ	RN, RN*, MD, U	RN, RN*-Bacc-Ed	Dist, DoE	X	X	Ed/CE
NM	LPN*, RN*, HD, MD	LPN*-exp, RN*	DoE	X		Competency
NY	RN, RN*, HD, MD, D, U	RN, RN-Ed, RN*-Bacc-Ed	Dist, DoH, DoE	X		Ed/CE
NC	RN	RN	Dist	X	X	NC
ND	LPN, RN, HD, MD, D, U	LPN, RN	Dist			
OH	RN*, HD, MD, D, U	RN*-Bacc-ed	DoE	X	X	
OK	LPN, RN, RN*, HD, U	RN*	DoE	X	X	
OR	RN, RN*, HD, MD, D	RN*-Bacc-Ed	DoE	X		Ed
PA	RN*, MD, D, U	RN*-BSN-Ed	DoE	X	X	Ed/CE
RI	RN, RN*, HD, MD, D, U	RN*-Bacc-Ed-exp	DoE	X	X	Ed, exp
SC	LPN, RN	LPN, RN	Dist			
SD	RN, HD, U	RN	Dist		X	
TN	LPN, RN, HD, MD, D, U	LPN, RN	Dist, DoH		X	
TX	LPN, RN, MD, U	RN	Dist	X		
UT	RN, HD, MD, D, U	RN	Dist			

(*continued*)

Table 3.1

State Regulations for School Nurse (SN) Practice (*continued*)

State	Authorized to Provide Health Services in Schools	Criteria for Becoming a SN	Source of Title	SN Protected Title	SN Mandate	Renewal Requirement
VT	RN*, HD, MD, D	RN*-Ed-exp, RN*-BSN-Ed-exp	DoE	X	X	Ed/CE
VA	LPN, RN, MD, U	RN*-Ed-exp, RN*-BSN-Ed-exp	DoE	X	X	Ed/CE
WA	RN, RN*, PHN, MD	RN*-Ed, RN*-BSN-Ed/exp	DoE	X		Ed/CE, exp
WV	LPN, RN*, HD, MD, D, U	RN*, RN*-BSN-Ed, RN*-MSN-NC	DoE	X	X	Ed, MS/age
WI	RN*, RN*, HD, MD, D	RN, RN*-BSN-Ed	Dist, DoE	X		Ed/CE if RN*
WY	RN*	RN*, RN-BSN	DoE	X		Ed/CE

Note: BoN = Board of Nursing; Bacc = baccalaureate; CE = continuing education learning experiences; D = dentist; Dist = local school district; DoE = Department of Education; DoH = Department of Health; Ed = formal or specific coursework; exp = experience; HD = health department staff; LPN = licensed practical or vocational nurse; MD = physician or chiropractor; NC = national certification, including National Board for Certification of School Nurses (NBCSN), American Nurses Credentialing Center (ANCC), and so on; PHN = public health nurse; RN = registered nurse; RN* = registered nurse credentialed as a school nurse in state; SN = school nurse; U = unlicensed person.

Source: Praeger, S., & Zimmerman, B. (2009). State regulations for school nurse practice. *Journal of School Nursing, 25*(6), 466–475. doi:10.1177/1059840509352655 (p. 469). Reprinted with permission from Sage Publications.

SCOPE OF PRACTICE, VARIABLES, AND SUBSPECIALTIES

Scope of Practice

Most school nurses work in a public school setting. However, the school nurse may also be employed to work in alternate sites such as residential settings, juvenile justice facilities, or occupational settings. Nurses may also provide services within the community that include after-school events, summer camps, field trips, or sporting events.

Variables

A school nurse's role can differ significantly, depending upon a number of variables. These include the following:

- *Grade level of students*: Prekindergarten, elementary, middle, or high school
- *Size of school*: Small (500 or fewer students), midsized (about 1,000 students), or large (more than 1,000 students)
- *Type of district*: Urban, suburban, or rural
- *Income level of community*: Low, middle, or high
- *Type of school*: Public, parochial, special needs, charter, or residential

Subspecialties

Considering the aforementioned numerous variables, subspecialties have developed that permit a higher level of expertise for a particular group. This specialization fosters even better care and greater understanding of needs. It is logical to expect that the nurse working with preschool-aged handicapped children will have quite a different job than the nurse at an urban high school. Subspecialties might include the following:

- Special needs
- Preschool
- Rural
- Urban
- Suburban
- High school
- Middle school
- Elementary school

Fast Facts

All school nurses must adapt to the individual needs of their students and community. Allow yourself the opportunity to explore different types of school settings. You may be surprised to learn that you have strengths you previously did not recognize.

(*continued*)

(continued)

Clinical Snapshot

School nurse Mary Beth was dismayed when she was assigned to the high school instead of the elementary school where a nurse had retired. Recognizing that the school district and superintendent had this option, she resigned herself to accepting the high school position. Several years later when Mary Beth was offered the elementary position, she decided to stay at the high school. Mary Beth found she enjoyed working with older students and honestly felt that this is where she was needed most.

THE FUTURE OF SCHOOL NURSING

It is doubtful that our school nurse pioneers ever imagined our profession would grow into what it is today. We can reasonably assume that the need for qualified nurses to care for children will continue to increase for the following reasons:

- Children are spending more time in school through participation in before- and after-school programs, sporting activities, school-sponsored trips, and so on. For many, the school nurse is their only source of medical attention.
- Infant survival has improved, and there are more multiple births. These infants frequently have problems at birth and present later in childhood with medical issues in school. The school nurse is needed to ensure their care.
- There are more children with chronic diseases and life-threatening allergies than ever before. School nurses must be available to meet their immediate needs.
- Today's educators now recognize that all children learn from each other. We no longer separate special needs children from their peers, but rather support the placement of children *in the least restrictive environment*. This is the law. School nurses are needed to assess these special children and monitor their medical needs in the academic setting. Therefore, they must be prepared to function at the highest level possible.

References

American Nurses Association and National Association of School Nurses. (2011). *School nursing: Scope and standards of practice* (2nd ed.). Silver Spring, MD: Nursebooks.org.

National Association of School Nurses. (2016a). *Education, licensure, and certification of School Nurses.* Retrieved from htpps://www.nasn.ort/advocacy/professional-practice-documents../ps-education
National Association of School Nurses. (2016b). *School nurse certification.* Retrieved from http://www.nasn.org/RoleCareer/SchoolNurseCertification
National Board for Certification of School Nurses. Certification Procedures. (2012). Retrieved from https://www.nbcsn.org
Praeger, S., & Zimmerman, B. (2009). State regulations for school nurse practice. *Journal of School Nursing, 25*(6), 466–475. doi:10.1177/1059840509352655
Schwab, N., & Gelfman, M. (Eds.). (2001). *Legal issues in school health services: A resource for school administrators, school attorneys and school nurses* (pp. 499–500). North Branch, MN: Sunrise River Press.

4

The School Health Office

After reading the previous chapters, you should have a greater understanding of, and respect for, school nurses and their role in the educational process. Now you are ready to set up the school health office and begin to work in your new home away from home.

The health office, its location, the way it is set up, and how the nurse interacts with students and faculty will establish the school nurse as either a totally insignificant entity or the "heart of the school."

In this chapter, you will learn:

1. Why the health office is an important part of the school
2. How to implement the six steps in the nursing process to assess students' needs
3. When to administer first aid and how to handle common illnesses and accidents
4. Mental illness and the school nurse's role in identifying and helping the student.

HEALTH OFFICE LOCATION

The health office should be centrally located and as close as possible to the gym, playground, lunchroom, and any room containing children with life-threatening conditions that could result in a classroom emergency. It must be well lit and ventilated. Air conditioning should be available as needed.

Newer schools were built with these specifications in mind. Many older school buildings were designed appropriately at the time of construction, but as student enrollments grew and more special-services personnel were required by law, the health office may have been moved to a less advantageous location. Making administrators aware of what constitutes a proper health office location may be your first and most difficult task.

Bathroom Facilities

A separate bathroom is essential. Ideally, you should have two sinks: one inside the bathroom and a clean sink outside the bathroom with an available eye wash station.

Fast Facts

Consider not providing a lock on the bathroom door. You *must* be able to enter immediately if a student becomes ill while in the bathroom.

Clinical Snapshot

Mrs. S., a long-time faculty member, prefers to use the health office bathroom, which is right next to her classroom, rather than go down the hall to the faculty lounge. She is upset that Darlene, the new school nurse, has had the lock on the bathroom door removed and insists on her privacy, indicating that *the previous nurse allowed a lock*. Darlene explains that this bathroom is for sick children and staff members only. She needs immediate access to anyone who is ill, and Mrs. S. would not want exposure to these germs. Darlene explains that this is her own decision and that it is nonnegotiable.

Health Office Space

A resting place should be available for children who become ill while at school. If space does not permit the separation of a child who is ill from other children, arrange for chairs or a bench to be placed outside the office where students can wait to see you. Leave your door open so that you can monitor them until you have tended to and secluded a child who is ill.

Creating a Warm and Caring Atmosphere

The atmosphere in your office should be warm and welcoming. Permit students and staff to feel that the school health office is a place of refuge. At the same time, avoid allowing any one individual or group to spend excessive amounts of time hanging around. This is not a place for faculty, parent, or student friends to gather and socialize. Your first responsibility is the students' health.

Once your office is arranged properly, you can begin the many other necessary tasks. *See Appendix B for more information regarding assessment tools, first-aid supplies, and other necessary equipment. Appendix C provides a suggested month-by-month calendar of tasks.*

Fast Facts

Make sure you and your desk are visible from the hall. There are students who will find comfort just knowing you are there in case they need you.

Clinical Snapshot

Lisa, a second grader, has become school phobic. Her parents recently divorced, and Mom has full custody. Lisa is fearful that, like her dad, Mom will also be gone when she comes home from school. School nurse Darlene arranges for Lisa to be left with her in the morning, and Darlene personally walks her to class. Lisa is permitted to pass the health office several times a day, and seeing Darlene, she is comforted.

Suggestions for Health Office Management

- Invite new students to visit your office when they are not ill. For the lower grades, have the teachers bring their class to you on the first day of school. Older students need assurance as well, so set aside time to meet them, and explain your role. Do not miss an opportunity to introduce yourself to new students and parents.
- Be careful whom you allow to use your phone, bathroom, and cot. Once you start permitting these privileges, it is difficult to stop.
- Learn to triage. You will quickly identify the students who are truly ill and those who just want to visit.

The nursing process "encompasses all significant actions taken by nurses in providing care to all clients, and forms the foundation for clinical decision making" (American Nurses Association, 2013). Whenever a student enters the health office, the school nurse must follow the appropriate steps of this process.

Five Steps of the School Nursing Process

1. *Assessment:* Note the child's complaint, take vital signs (temperature, pulse, respiration [TPR], blood pressure [BP]) and a history of the complaint, and examine as needed. Do not forget to include the fifth vital sign: pain assessment: location, duration, intensity (use 1–10 scale or face chart if nonverbal).
2. *Diagnosis:* Formulate a diagnosis, based on the assessment data collected.
3. *Planning:* Develop a plan of care or action for the child.
4. *Implementation:* Implement the intervention identified; return the child to class, or exclude him or her from school.
5. *Evaluation:* Evaluate the outcome of the plan; follow up by checking on the student at an appropriate time.

FIRST AID

Regardless of the time of day or evening, when you are in the school building, you are on duty. No other nurse will give you a report at the beginning of your shift, and what you do not finish one day will be waiting for you when you return to the school health office. Every student, staff member, and visitor to the school is your potential patient. You may also be asked to be available for school-sponsored activities, such as sporting events and overnight trips. No two days will be the same, and first aid must be the task you tend to before all others.

Fast Facts

Watch the *frequent flyers!* Try to establish an understanding that if a child just wishes to visit, he or she can come at an appropriate time, for example, during recess, during lunch, or before or after school. The child does not need to invent an illness. This way when he or she is truly ill, you will be less likely to overlook it. Frequent flyer or not, follow the nursing process.

Clinical Snapshot

First-grader Michael comes to school nurse Darlene, complaining that he has a headache. Darlene follows the nursing process to assess him. Michael is pale and appears tired: His temperature is 97.8°F, pulse is 100, and blood pressure is 100/60 mmHg. Darlene asks how long he has had the headache and whether he has eaten

(*continued*)

(continued)

breakfast (*assessment*). She allows Michael to rest for 10 minutes, noting his body language and how he interacts with other children coming in and out of the office. Michael seems fine (*diagnosis*) after resting, but since he seldom comes to see Darlene, she sends a note to the teacher, asking her to observe and refer back if Michael is unable to do his work (*outcome*). Darlene checks on Michael at lunchtime (*plan*), and he tells her his headache is better, but she notes he did not finish his lunch. She rechecks his temperature and tells him to let her know if the headache returns (*implementation*). She leaves a message at home, alerting Michael's parents of his earlier complaint and poor appetite, and asks that they check him again in the evening (*evaluation*).

This is where your previous experience will come into play. Learning to prioritize tasks is essential; with practice, you will become proficient.

Standing Orders

All school districts should be operating under medical standing orders. These orders are basic guidelines that govern how you are to render first aid. They are based on state codes and are generated by the school nurse and approved, in writing, by the school physician.

Standing orders should be the same throughout a school district and updated annually. If your district does not have standing orders or the procedures are disorganized, work with your district colleagues and school physician to formulate and standardize them. You can solicit samples from other districts and adapt them for your use. Make sure you inform your principal, in writing, that developing standing orders is a mandated task necessary to protect your license and the school district. Share the final product with your principal.

Assessment

All students who seek you out must be appropriately assessed using the nursing process. (For very young students, you may need to speak with parents or teachers to obtain accurate histories.) Most standing orders for rendering first aid are organized into categories: acute illnesses, chronic illnesses, accidents, and behavioral issues. Some common illnesses and basic guidelines to help you properly assess students follow.

Acute Illnesses

Typical acute illnesses of school-age children include viral infections, bacterial infections, rashes, skin lesions, respiratory infections, headaches, and stomachaches.

General Treatment for Acute Illnesses

- Check vital signs, look at the child's throat and ears, listen to breath sounds, and feel the abdomen.
- Watch body language; note skin appearance.
- Take the history of the complaint: When did the pain start? Did the child eat breakfast? When did he or she last urinate or have a bowel movement? Was he or she ill during the night? What was he or she doing in class when the pain started?
- Notify a parent. Exclude the child from class if necessary, or tell the parent that you will be checking on the child periodically and that he or she should expect a return call if the child's condition does not improve.
- If these factors are insignificant, keep the child for a short observation period, then allow the child to return to class, and recheck the child in an hour, or exclude from school.

Chronic Illnesses

Some common chronic illnesses of the school-age child include allergies, asthma, diabetes, cardiac conditions, tuberculosis, and seizure disorders.

Fast Facts

It is the goal of the school health program to recognize students' chronic conditions and manage manifestations in school. Unless absolutely necessary, chronically ill children should *not* be excluded because of restrictions secondary to their illnesses. Plans should be in place to control symptoms as they arise so the child can return to class.

Clinical Snapshot

Asthmatic children present a special challenge to school nurses. David, grade 6, needs to take his inhaler before gym class. He is competent in its use and may self-administer. School nurse Darlene wrote an individualized healthcare plan and emergency

(*continued*)

(continued)

care plan for his care. Darlene informed David's classroom and physical education teachers of his needs and arranged for him to have a nebulizer with his personal medication available. Darlene is trained in airway management and will not hesitate to summon help if needed.

General Treatment for Chronic Illnesses

Have an individualized healthcare plan (IHP) and an emergency care plan (ECP) in place for each child to address his or her specific condition. The plans should be written by the school nurse in concert with the student, parent(s), physician, teachers, and administrator. They contain the nursing diagnosis, student goals, interventions, evaluation, and specific instructions in the event of an emergency. Plans provided for chronic conditions must include, at a minimum, the following information:

- *Allergies:* The allergen, preventive measures for exposure, and epinephrine autoinjector availability
- *Asthma:* An asthma action plan, medication availability, and nebulizer treatments
- *Diabetes:* Snack and exercise schedule, blood glucose testing times, glucagon and other medication needs
- *Cardiac condition:* The nature of the illness and restrictions
- *Tuberculosis:* The medication regimen and follow-up monitoring
- Medication use and oxygen availability

Accidents

Common school accidents include fractures, eye injuries, lacerations, burns, and skull and dental trauma. If severe, do not hesitate to send for an ambulance.

General Treatment for Accidents

- *Fractures:* If deformity is apparent or skin is broken, cover with sterile gauze, then apply splints and ice.
- *Eye injuries:* For a foreign body, rinse at the eye station. If the object is not dislodged, loosely cover the eye, and refer the person to a physician. For all other eye trauma, refer immediately.
- *Lacerations:* Cleanse, apply a dressing, and refer those with facial and large lacerations to a physician.

- *Burns:* Apply a cool compress; do no break blisters. Call an ambulance if the area involved is large and you suspect a third-degree burn.
- *Head trauma:* Do not move the person; check for bleeding and orientation. Call an ambulance. Head injuries have received increased attention recently. It was once thought that a child's developing brain was more likely to recover fully after an injury because it was flexible and would rewire over time. However, there is now more evidence that deficits manifest years later when the brain is mature and a higher level of reasoning is expected (Brain Injury Association of America, 2004). In all cases involving head trauma, you *must* do the following:
  - Document incidents in and out of school on the permanent health record.
  - Support you school's policy on sports participation following head trauma. If you feel strongly that it should be tightened, make your concerns known in writing to the school physician and administration.
  - Carefully assess every child: Have the child lie down, check pupils, and so on.
  - Notify parents even for seemingly minor head injuries.
- *Dental trauma:* Save any teeth in a preservative or the injured person's saliva; refer to a dentist.

Fast Facts

For situations requiring an ambulance, have the student transported to the closest medical facility. Do *not* wait for parents to arrive at the school. Situations in which an ambulance is definitely needed include:

Suspected or actual anaphylaxis	Head trauma
Airway obstruction or respiratory distress	Large skin burn
Cardiac arrest	Open fracture

Clinical Snapshot

Catherine's mother is a nurse at the regional medical center several towns away. Mom indicates that Catherine is to be taken *only* to her hospital, not the local one closest to the school. School nurse Darlene discusses this in advance and clarifies with her that all emergencies must be treated as such and transferred to the *closest facility.* Once there, parents can sign out and transfer their child wherever they wish.

Behavioral Issues

Behavioral issues can include school phobia, tantrums, depression, and anxiety disorders. Frequently, the school nurse becomes involved in helping students who are experiencing separation issues or emotional problems. Beware of the frequent visitor. It is easy to miss a true illness in a child who sees you every day with minor complaints.

General Treatment for Behavioral Issues

- Communicate closely with the student, parent(s), and teachers.
- Develop a plan.
- Refer to specific professional help, and remain available.

MENTAL HEALTH

Mental health can be conceptualized as a state of well-being in which the individual realized his or her own abilities, can cope with the normal stresses of life, can work productively and fruitfully, and is able to make a contribution to his or her community.

World Health Organization (2014)

There are a number of reasons why the school nurse must be alert and responsive to mental health issues in the school setting.

- Mental health issues are very common. Depression, anxiety, and substance abuse are seen in all children and adults.
- Most people are completely incapable of recognizing a mental health issue and responding appropriately. Mental health first aid focuses on identifying, understanding, and responding to signs of mental illness. Usually there are warning signs. Once we are alerted to them, it is our responsibility to assess the level of concern and risk for suicide and refer immediately for professional help.
- The school nurse can play an important role in listening to each child's complaint nonjudgmentally.
- There remains a stigma associated with mental illness, and many will never seek help. When they do seek help, frequently, it is not available. The school nurse can provide appropriate contacts for the distressed child or adult.

Under *no* circumstances should you:

1. Permit yourself to take on the role of counselor. This is not your job, nor are you trained to do so.

2. Promise not to share information. If the situation is dire, report to appropriate personnel.
3. Allow the child/adult to go home to an unsafe environment.
4. Share any information with other staff and parents unless there is an obvious reason for them to know.

Role of School Nurses in Rendering First Aid

- *You* make the assessment. Do not be influenced by teachers or parents.
- Assess every child who enters your office. Remain calm and confident.
- Discourage students, parents, and colleagues from coming to school for you to diagnose when they are ill. You are not a physician.
- If you are uncertain whether a child should be sent home or to the hospital in an ambulance, call 911. *Always err on the side of caution.*
- Learn to triage, and remain current on all first-aid procedures.
- Prominently display in your office and on your phone the emergency numbers and names of other people in your school who are certified in cardiopulmonary resuscitation and use of an automated external defibrillator.
- Call the child's parent(s) for even minor issues. This allows the parent(s) to decide whether to ignore the problem, come into school immediately to evaluate the child themselves, or deal with a situation at home.
- When asked for a physician referral, offer the names of several local doctors. Allow parents to choose for themselves.
- Have accurate, updated emergency contact information available for every child and adult in your building.

Resources

Mental Health First Aid: https://www.mentalhealthfirstaid.org/

Nursing Process: Purpose and Steps: https://study.com/academy/lesson/nursing-process-purpose-and-steps.html

What Is Nursing & What Do Nurses Do? | ANA Enterprise: https://www.nursingworld.org/practice-policy/workforce/what-is-nursing/

References

American Nurses Association. (2013). *The nursing process steps.* Retrieved from https://www.nursingworld.org/practice-policy/workforce/what-is-nursing/the-nursing-process/

Brain Injury Association of America. (2004). *Brain injury in children.* Retrieved from https://www.biausa.org/brain-injury/about-brain-injury/children-what-to-expect

World Health Organization. (2014). *Mental Health: Strengthening our response* (Fact Sheet No 220). Retrieved from http://www.who.int/mediacentre/factsheets/fs220/en/

II

Health Appraisal in School Nursing: Health Promotion and Disease Prevention

5

The Big Three: Immunizations, Screenings, and Medications

Monitoring immunizations, performing screenings, and administering medications are three of the major areas in school nursing practice for which we are totally responsible. We are the gatekeepers for maintaining school compliance for all immunizations; detecting, referring, and following up on vision, hearing, height, weight, blood pressure, and scoliosis through mass screenings; and giving medications so students can remain in school and function at their highest level of wellness.

The big three *represent our overwhelming responsibility to children, our employers, and our profession.*

In this chapter, you will learn:

1. The school nurse's responsibility in immunization monitoring
2. Basic elements of the screening process
3. General guidelines for administering medications

IMMUNIZATIONS

The control of communicable diseases was one of the original reasons for placing nurses in school settings and remains a major responsibility of school nurses today. Administrators depend on school nurses to uphold health regulations and to keep them informed of any deficiencies. Every state has specific legislation regarding immunizations.

Fast Facts

Every state has immunization requirements for children who attend school. It is imperative that you know your state and district policies regarding immunization requirements, the parental rights of refusal, and the reportable infectious diseases.

Clinical Snapshot

David recently transferred into the school where Samantha is the nurse. Records from his previous out-of-state school indicate that he is in full compliance with all required immunizations. However, her state requires additional immunizations. The different policy must be explained to the parents, and David should be permitted to attend school while receiving the remaining required immunizations.

Some parents question the safety of the numerous vaccines required today and mistrust or resist government requirements. These parents have a right to express their concerns to you. However, if too large a number of parents refuses immunizations for their children, preventable diseases will re-emerge and cause illnesses and deaths, as they have in the past. For the overall health of all students, it is imperative that all be fully immunized according to state public health requirements. The recommended immunizations for children from birth through 6 years of age and 7 through 18 years of age can be found on the Centers for Disease Control and Prevention (CDC) website: https://www.cdc.gov/vaccines/schedules/index.html.

Generally, you may accept immunization documentation from the following sources:

- A private physician: A signed certificate, prescription, or note with letterhead
- A public health department: Official record
- A previous school: Official school or child care records
- Each entry must contain the complete date (month, day, and year)

Healthy People 2020 Objectives: Immunization and Infectious Diseases, 19: Increase the number of states collecting kindergarten vaccine coverage data according to the CDC minimum standards from 13 in 2009 to 51 (including the District of Columbia).

Fast Facts

Be aware that many countries list the day first and then the month and year. For example, an immunization given in the United States on December 2, 2002, would be recorded as 12/2/2002; the same date could be recorded internationally as 02/12/2002.

Clinical Snapshot

School nurse Samantha had to translate the recorded birth date for a student from the United Kingdom and then recheck all the dates of the immunizations to make sure vaccines were given at the appropriate ages and intervals according to her state's laws.

You may encounter parents who have not had their children immunized for a variety of reasons, including strong religious or philosophical beliefs, fear, indifference, or ignorance. Parents are not forced to make a decision regarding immunization until their children enter school and the governing laws demand compliance before admission. This can be a difficult situation. Be sympathetic, yet firm, and stress that you are implementing a state law.

Contraindications for Immunizations

Medical

All states permit medical exclusions, although exemptions may vary. It is not required to give a child any immunization that is medically contraindicated. Requests for exemption must state the reason and the period of time for which immunization is to be withheld, and they must be signed by a physician or, where permitted, an advanced practice registered nurse and reviewed annually.

Religious

If a required immunization conflicts with the student's religious beliefs or practices, the parents must request the exemption in writing. The document must state how the vaccine conflicts with their religious beliefs or practices. A copy of the document should be forwarded to your administrator for legal review. This is *not* the same as a philosophical, moral, or conscientious exemption.

Philosophical

Eighteen states permit philosophical exemptions. These states do not restrict the exemptions to purely religious or spiritual beliefs. Their objection may be based on moral, philosophical, or other personal beliefs (National Conference of State Legislatures, 2017). For a complete list of all states' permitted exclusions, visit the Immunization Action Coalition website (www.immunize.org/laws/exemptions.asp).

Provisional

A child may be allowed to attend school after he or she has received an initial dose of the required immunization and is in the process of completing the series. Parents must keep you updated as immunizations are given.

Role of School Nurses in Meeting Immunization Requirements

- Strongly recommend that all health information be submitted *before* children enter school. Get administrative support to exclude those who are noncompliant.
- Review any new student's information: Registration form, health history, physical examination, immunizations received, previous school records, emergency card, and so on.
- Document dates on each permanent health record and review annually, noting any recent changes in requirements.
- Refer back to the physician or clinic for deficiencies.
- Recheck *all* students' immunizations for deficiencies at least annually.
- Review and update students' records with medical, religious, philosophical, and provisional status.
- Know your state's immunization regulations. File the immunization status report as required in your state, and allow local or state officials access to your files for the purposes of audit or survey.
- Be cautious with noncompliant parents. Refer back to private physicians for reassurances as to safety.

Fast Facts

Until a child reaches the age when he or she is required by law to attend school, parents can choose not to immunize their child. If that is the case, you will be the first one to confront the parent with the law.

Clinical Snapshot

Mr. and Mrs. K. register their twin boys in May for kindergarten. School nurse Samantha notes that neither has received any immunizations.

(*continued*)

(continued)

Both parents are adamant that their children *not* receive immunizations or *any foreign substance in their bodies.* Samantha states that although she believes in the importance of protecting children from disease, she respects their rights as parents. She informs the parents that she is serving as an agent of the board of education and must act according to the laws of the state and district. Samantha agrees to work with them and provide steps they must take to resolve the issue. Samantha explains that they can seek a medical or religious exemption and describes the process involved. She remains nonjudgmental and forwards all information to the principal for the school attorney to review.

SCREENINGS

Screenings are considered the secondary level of prevention. The goal is early detection and prompt treatment of deficiencies *before* they become health problems. When children are screened, those with no obvious problem are separated from those who need to be seen by a physician.

Role of School Nurses in the Screening Process

- Know the district and state laws relevant to screening in the school setting.
- Have all equipment calibrated and in good working condition; know how to use it.
- Obtain necessary written permission from parents according to school policy.
- Know the grade levels, previous referrals, and special students who must be screened yearly.
- Seek cooperation from staff to arrange for students to be screened at mutually convenient times.

Fast Facts

You may choose to do all your screenings individually or allot a certain amount of time per student and do all the screenings at once. Do what works best for you and is the least disruptive for the

(continued)

(*continued*)

students and teachers. States vary significantly in the number and types of required health screenings.

Clinical Snapshot

School nurse Samantha schedules each child for a 10-minute block of time when performing mandated screenings. She sends for three students at a time, has them bring material to read while waiting, and performs all screenings—vision, hearing, height, weight, blood pressure, and scoliosis—during this visit. Samantha enjoys this time with each child and the opportunity to talk with them individually.

Samantha's colleagues prefer to do each screening separately. They feel this provides an opportunity to see every student at least several times throughout the school year, and not just those who are *frequent flyers*.

- Using the guidelines recommended by your school physician, make referrals after you have checked several times or immediately if you find a defect that is profound.
- Document findings on worksheets; transfer them to the permanent record.
- Follow up on all referrals to see that care is rendered.
- Let parents know that if they do not hear from you, they may assume their child passed the screening.
- Recheck all students who fail the initial screening at least once before sending out a referral.

Fast Facts

Be sensitive to the child's right to privacy. Do *not* announce the child's weight or any other information for others to hear.

Clinical Snapshot

Samantha makes certain that students cannot see the scale numbers and refuses to tell any child what they weigh while she is screening them. She tells students to see her after school if they wish to know the numbers.

Fast Facts

Ask your administrator to allow you to screen without interruptions. Request that the principal designate someone to handle nonurgent issues.

Clinical Snapshot

Samantha informed the office secretary and principal of the times she and the classroom teachers had agreed upon for screenings. She was interrupted three times during the first 30 minutes to attend to a child with an upset stomach, a student who wanted to use the phone to call home for sneakers, and a child with a nosebleed that had stopped by the time Samantha got to him. Samantha had to explain the importance of this time for proper assessment and asked that she should only be disturbed for an *emergency.* Samantha then defined an emergency.

If the interruptions continue, Samantha should request a substitute to cover her office while she is screening students.

Typical School Screenings for All Students

Blood pressure
Dental
Drug
Hearing
Height, weight, body mass index
Scoliosis
Tuberculosis
Vision

Fast Facts

Consider planning your screenings according to the season. The few minutes you save in attending to each child add up.

Clinical Snapshot

Samantha schedules height and weight screenings at the beginning of the school year so she can see and talk with every student

(continued)

(continued)

and identify immediate problems. She tries to complete all the hearing screenings before the temperature drops and the cold season begins, knowing that head congestion will interfere with a reliable result. Samantha holds off on blood pressure screening until the spring, when children are more likely to wear short sleeves; this allows for quicker cuff placement.

MEDICATIONS

Administration of medications, both prescribed and over the counter, is an area of high risk and can be extremely difficult for the school nurse. Because of the large number of students with chronic health conditions and disabilities, often there is no choice but to medicate while at school. The nurse has an obligation to ensure that the procedure for safe dispensing is closely followed.

Accept medications from an adult only in original containers that indicate clearly the student's name, medication, dosage, and times to be given. Epinephrine and inhalers must be kept accessible, but all other medications should be locked, including those refrigerated. Controlled substances should be counted in the presence of an adult and kept secure in a double-locked cabinet.

Most school policies demand an annual written order from a physician or advanced practice registered nurse and a signed parental consent to dispense medications. Standardized forms for this purpose are usually available for parents and physicians to use.

People Authorized to Give Medication in School

School policies usually permit only the following people to dispense medications:

- The school physician
- A certified or noncertified nurse employed by the district
- A substitute school nurse employed by the district
- A student's parent or guardian
- A student who is approved to self-administer in certain life-threatening conditions, such as anaphylaxis or asthma
- School employees trained and delegated to administer medication in emergencies

Fast Facts

Do not make exceptions for *anyone* regarding routine medication administration. Stick to the official policy, for your protection and that of the district.

Clinical Snapshot

School nurse Samantha worked for years in a hospital setting. She knew of numerous nurses who had made medication errors. Typically, the first reported error was handled by a warning. If a second occurred, the nurse would be sent for a remedial lesson on medication administration. The third error would result in termination. Schools are quite different. That first error could mean your job. Be cautious, and stick to your district policy.

Epinephrine, Glucagon, Naloxone, and Diastat Administration and Delegate Training

Schools are required to have policies in place to deal with anaphylactic reactions for diagnosed and undiagnosed children with life-threatening allergies or diagnoses. It is your responsibility to have the medication available and to train delegates to recognize symptoms and use the proper technique to administer the injection.

Many states also have regulations permitting glucagon, naloxone, or Diastat administration by noncertified personnel. You will be responsible for delegate training for these individuals as well.

Field Trips

If a child requires medication at any school-sponsored event, nursing coverage may be required. A policy must be in place and a substitute nurse hired to attend the event.

Types of Medications Given at School

Behavior Modification

Today, many of these drugs are given once a day at home. You may offer to keep one dose available in case a parent calls to tell you that a dose was missed at home. You must still have an order from the physician and written parental consent.

Antibiotics

Unless written in a healthcare plan, administer only if the medication is ordered three or four times a day.

Emergencies

- Asthma: oral inhalers, nebulizers
- Epinephrine, Benadryl, glucagon, Diastat

Fast Facts

There are numerous gray areas in the practice of school nursing. Do not hesitate to send the ill child home, call an ambulance, or uphold your medication policy. This may mean that you are not loved by everyone, but that is okay.

Clinical Snapshot

Samantha replaced a beloved school nurse who had worked in the same location for 25 years. Samantha constantly meets resistance to any change she attempts. Samantha will need to learn to choose her battles, compromise when she can, and be forceful when necessary in hopes that in time she will be appreciated for the contribution she makes to the school.

Role of School Nurses in Medication Administration

- Know your district policy on medications and follow it exactly. If you disagree with how it is written, get clarification before it becomes an issue.
- According to the Food and Drug Administration, herbal remedies and food supplements are *not* considered medications and should not be given at school.
- Avoid giving medications in school whenever possible. Medications ordered once or twice a day can be taken at home.
- It is preferable for the first and second doses of antibiotics be given at home in case of a reaction.
- Carefully document the medication given for each student.
- Have physicians' orders and signed parental consents updated yearly.
- Permit students to self-administer according to state regulations and school policy.

- Train delegates to administer emergency medications as permitted by state regulations and school policy.

Reference

National Conference of State Legislatures. (2017). Retrieved from http://www.ncsl.org/research/health/school-immunization-exemption-state-laws.aspx

6

Student Health Assessments

Starting sometime in early May, parents initiate the "school crusade" on behalf of their children. They insist on certain teachers and arrangements for the upcoming fall classes. Then comes the flood of July advertisements for school clothes, sneakers, backpacks, and other paraphernalia that parents purchase to ensure that their children have the essential tools for success in school.

Yet these same conscientious parents may never consider scheduling routine health examinations for their children. They may give no thought to whether their children are physically and emotionally ready for school and capable of fully participating in the academic and sports programs. This is where the school nurse steps in.

In this chapter, you will learn:

1. Why periodic health assessments are essential to learning
2. When is the most appropriate time for students to be assessed
3. The rationale for adolescent depression screening
4. Why chronic absenteeism is so harmful
5. Major reasons for poor school attendance
6. The history and pros and cons of school-based clinics

STUDENT HEALTH ASSESSMENTS

Physical examinations for school children began as far back as 1920. Their purpose was to identify children with "defects" (Wold, 1981), with the rationale that no student's learning potential should be compromised by a remediable physical disability and that every student should be free of communicable diseases and be able to participate fully in all school activities. The examinations were done at school or by private physicians.

Critics argued that examinations performed at school were too costly and superficial; without parental input, there could be no complete detection of health problems.

Beginning around 1950, most required examinations were performed by private physicians in their offices. These examinations were more comprehensive than those that had been performed at school but proved to be costly in time and money for the parents. Often, students were noncompliant, and districts were left with the difficult decision of whether such children should be excluded from school, physical education class, or sports.

Fast Facts

Today, school examinations are referred to as health assessments because subjective and objective information must be gathered and interpreted by the health professional. The entire body, from head to toe, is considered, as is a child's emotional wellness.

Clinical Snapshot

School nurse Joan frequently checks with the parents of children she knows have emotional issues. If she is aware that a student has been absent for a prolonged period or is suffering from depression, she initiates a call giving a heads-up about any potential problem and inquires how the student is doing at home.

All schools require physical assessments according to state law or local district policy. They may vary in frequency and depth. Most districts offer assessments in school or will help to arrange free clinic visits for students. Assessments are performed by physicians or advanced practice nurses.

Types of Assessments

School nurses are concerned with two types of assessments: routine wellness and athletic assessments.

Routine Assessments

Routine assessments can be required of students:

- Upon entrance to school within a specified period of time (usually 1 year)
- During the early childhood years (grades K–3)
- During preadolescence (grades 4–6)
- Upon reaching adolescence (grades 7–12)
- When referred for child study team evaluation
- When applying for work permits
- When suspected of drug abuse

A routine assessment must note any health problems and state clearly whether the student may or may not participate in physical education classes. It must identify any physical education restrictions, and if it is conducted at school, parental consent must be obtained in writing. A physician-signed, standardized form is commonly used.

Athletic Assessments

Most school districts now have specific procedures and forms for participation in athletics. Assessments and questionnaires usually must be completed within a certain time frame before a sport begins. An athletic assessment includes, at minimum, the following components:

- A detailed health history, signed by the parent or guardian, which covers previous injuries, surgeries, loss of consciousness, and so on
- A comprehensive physical examination, including blood and urine analyses
- A statement from the examining physician permitting the student to participate
- Provisions for updates throughout the school year for other sports
- Written permission from the parent for the student to be examined and participate in the sport
- School-physician approval for all private-physician clearances

Depression Screening

The American Academy of Pediatrics now recommends that adolescents aged 10 to 21 years be screened for depression by their primary care clinicians. This recommendation is in response to the report by Dr. Zuckerbrot that cites that 50% of adolescents with depression are diagnosed before they reach adulthood and as many as two in three depressed teens do not get any help or care (Zuckerbrot, 2018).

Role of School Nurses in Assessments

- Know, understand, and implement the policies and procedures for the district.

- Scrutinize physical examination reports, noting any restrictions. Upon a physician's order or for any student not cleared in writing, exclude the student from participation in physical education classes and athletic competitions.
- Provide physical education teachers and coaches with a list of students who may not participate.
- Carefully document the results of all assessments on the permanent health record.
- If an assessment is done in school, provide necessary equipment and assistance.
- Add depression screening to your forms for physician completion. Follow up for results, especially if concerned about a particular student.
- Advocate for children. If you believe that participation in athletics is not in a child's best interest, put it in writing.

Chronic Absenteeism

A new analysis from the U.S. Department of Education (2016) reveals the following:

- Chronic absenteeism is prevalent throughout the country and includes all races as well as students with disabilities.
- Chronic absenteeism is characterized by a student's absence of 15 or more days in a school year.
- More than 6 million or 13% of all students missed at least 15 days of school in the 2013–2014 school year.
- High school students were absent the most (almost 20%), followed by middleschool (12%), and elementary students (10%).

"Chronic absenteeism is a national problem," said U.S. Secretary of Education John B. King Jr. "Frequent absences from school can be devastating to a child's education. Missing school leads to low academic achievement and triggers drop outs. Millions of young people are missing opportunities in postsecondary education, good careers and a chance to experience the American dream." (U.S. Department of Education, 2016)

Problems Associated With Frequent Absenteeism

- Chronic health conditions (asthma, cancer, etc.)
- Poverty
- Frequent family moves
- Unrest at home
- Feelings of isolation or not being connected with school
- Gaps in learning, especially in lower grades that provide the foundation for math and reading

Children with prolonged and frequent absences are at risk for failure in school. These children may choose to drop out altogether. Students are much more likely to succeed in school when they attend consistently. In addition, school budgets may suffer when absentee rates are high. State and federal funds may be awarded to schools that have low absentee rates, providing more money for essential classroom needs.

ATTENDANCE

According to law, every child is entitled to a free public education. To get such an education, a student must be well enough to learn and attend school consistently.

Fast Facts

Every child should be accounted for every day. This does not mean that nurses themselves need to make calls to check on absences. This should be the responsibility of office staff. The school nurse must be in touch with seriously ill children and follow up with those who are sent home.

Clinical Snapshot

As did her predecessor, school nurse Joan spends almost the entire morning handling attendance problems. However, Joan's job now also includes teaching two classes of health education a day, and she is becoming increasingly frustrated. She hates leaving her office when the attendance is incomplete and resents tracking down parents who do not call in. When she spoke with the principal, he said there was no one else to perform this clerical task. Nonetheless, Joan began to document the hours spent on attendance, and once the waste of professional time was itemized, the principal and Joan reached a compromise. The secretary would handle routine absences, and Joan would follow up on serious illnesses and accidents.

Fast Facts

All too often, children who are homeschooled or placed out of the district fall through the cracks. Remember, these are still your students. Your district is paying for a service in another school. The greater the number of people who monitor the child, the safer he or

(*continued*)

(*continued*)

she will be. You have a place in this process, especially if the placement is for a medical need. Maintain contact with the parents and the school nurse in the out-of-district school.

Clinical Snapshot

Mrs. K. has three children. The youngest, Amy, has special needs that require placement in a regional special education program. On a day when the rest of the staff is attending a math in-service program, school nurse Joan requests and receives permission to visit Amy at her school. Joan spends time in the classroom, talking with Amy and her teacher. She then stops in to see the school nurse. Joan is more than pleased with the care Amy is receiving and tells Mrs. K. Joan also suggests to the child study team that Amy be permitted to join her grade-level peers for special events in her school. Mrs. K. is appreciative and thanks her for not forgetting her child and for fostering inclusion.

Role of School Nurses in Monitoring Attendance

- Know your students, learn why they are absent, and, if possible, try to remedy the problem.
- Do not forget the children placed out of district or homeschooled. They are still your students.
- Monitor students who are frequently tardy or absent.
- Review and enforce the school policy on absenteeism.
- Control contagious diseases as much as possible: Exclude ill students from school, discourage acutely ill students from returning to school too quickly, and send notices home, informing parents of any widespread illnesses.
- Encourage healthful habits: Frequent handwashing, cleanliness, room ventilation, adequate rest and exercise, and proper nutrition. Be proactive in keeping your students healthy.
- Work to identify the true cause of absenteeism before a child is penalized unfairly.

Healthy People 2020 Objectives: Access to Health Services, 5.2:
Increase the proportion of children and youth aged 17 years and under who have a specific source of ongoing care from 94.3 in 2008 to 100%.

SCHOOL-BASED CLINICS

In the mid-1960s, during President Johnson's War on Poverty, it was noted that poor children in the United States were medically underserved. The establishment of Medicaid in 1965 increased the focus on the plight of low-income families. Because children were required to spend many hours a day at school, it was felt that schools were the logical place to provide the care offered by Medicaid. The rationale was as follows:

- Schools were more convenient and comfortable for students, especially in dealing with mental health issues. Health education could be directly targeted to those in need.
- Many families had inadequate or no health insurance, leaving children with few options for medical treatment.
- Schools dealt with many medically fragile students. On-site care was thought to be most beneficial.

Opponents of school-based clinics argued the following points:

- Children should not be given information about birth control at the clinics. Some felt that this would do little to affect risky sexual behavior.
- Funding was difficult. Multiple sources of income were necessary and not always forthcoming.

In 1986, the Robert Wood Johnson Foundation launched an adolescent healthcare program. It awarded grants up to $600,000 each to public and private schools in poor, overcrowded urban areas to set up adolescent healthcare centers. One of the grant criteria was that the staff of these clinics were to cooperate with school nurses, teachers, coaches, counselors, and school principals and their staffs.

The clinics were required to provide a comprehensive range of services, including the following:

- Treatment for common illnesses and minor injuries
- Referrals and follow-up for serious illnesses and emergencies
- On-site care and consultations, and follow-up for pregnancies
- Counseling and referrals for drug and alcohol abuse, sexual abuse, and risks of suicide
- On-site care and referrals for sexually transmitted infections
- Sports and employment physicals
- Immunizations (Keeton, Soleimanpour, & Brindis, 2012)

The 2013–2014 census done by the School Based Health Alliance showed there are currently 2,315 school-based health clinics (SBHCs) that serve students and communities in 49 of 50 states and the District of Columbia. The number of SBHCs nationally grew 20% since the

2011 census, with 385 new programs recognized in the Alliance's database (National Assembly School Based Alliance, 2018).

Thousands of students are now served by nurse practitioners and part-time physicians working in concert with the school nurse. Many more could benefit from this type of healthcare delivery.

Fast Facts

Providing all students with appropriate healthcare is a challenge. Suspect financial difficulties when medical forms are not returned. Assist families to find services, and follow through until their needs are met.

Clinical Snapshot

School nurse Joan is well aware of the families in her district that have low income levels and receive healthcare through the clinic of the local hospital. She does *not* always know of the family going through temporary tough times. She should suspect there is a financial problem when a parent is compliant with all school health requirements except those that cost money.

ROLE OF SCHOOL NURSES IN SCHOOL-BASED CLINICS

- Establish open lines of communication between the school health office and the local clinic. Remember, you both have the same goals.
- Refer students as needed.
- Remain diligent in protecting students' rights and privacy.
- If you are in a district where students' health needs are not being met, seek a remedy. Explore the possibility of a school-based clinic.

References

Keeton, V., Soleimanpour, S., & Brindis, C. D. (2012). School-based health centers in an era of health care reform: Building on history. *Current Problems in Pediatric and Adolescent Health Care, 42*(6), 132–158. doi:10.1016/j.cppeds.2012.03.002.

National Assembly School-Based Health Alliance. Retrieved from www.sbh4all.org/school-health-care/national-census-of-school-based-health-centers/

U.S. Department of Education. (2016, June 10). New data show chronic absenteeism is widespread and prevalent among all age groups. Retrieved from https://www.ed.gov/news/press-releases/new-data-show-chronic-absenteeism-widespread-and-prevalent-among-all-student-groups

Wold, S. J. (1981). *School nursing: A framework for practice* (pp. 3–17, 20–29, 39–47). North Branch, MN: Sunrise River Press.

Zuckerbrot, R. A., Cheung, A., Jensen, P. A. , Stein, R. E. K., & Laraque, D. L. (2018). Guidelines for adolescent depression in primary care (GLAD-PC): Part I. Practice preparation, identification, assessment, and initial management. *Pediatrics, 141*(3), 1–23. doi:10.1542/peds.2017-4081

7

Health Education

It has long been recognized that the most influential factor in a child's ability to learn is the teacher(s). Health, more than any other discipline, must be taught by well-qualified professionals who know the content and are comfortable with it. When that teacher has extensive, practical knowledge in the field and has already demonstrated a strong commitment to students, it is definitely a winning combination.

The school nurse is the perfect health educator; he or she has a strong medical background, is current on health issues, and is deeply devoted to children. With one foot in nursing and the other in education, the school nurse is the ideal person to identify, teach, and demonstrate healthful habits.

Health education is at the very core of the thrust toward primary prevention. Nurses teach instinctively every day of their professional lives, sometimes before a large group but more often informally, with the same good outcome.

In this chapter, you will learn:

1. The definition of *health education* and its function as a separate discipline
2. Risk factors for young people
3. Key elements of the *2017 National Youth Risk Behavior Surveillance Report*
4. The national standards for health education
5. The content of health education
6. How to teach health and health literacy
7. Obstacles to teaching health education

HEALTH EDUCATION

Definition

Health education is the totality of experiences that influence knowledge of, and attitudes toward, health. It should be meaningful to the learners, motivate them to maintain and improve their health, and provide them with the knowledge and skills they need in order to be healthy for a lifetime.

Health education has functioned as a separate discipline for a number of decades. However, it is still considered a relatively new discipline and struggles for a sense of identity (Gilbert, 2000, p. 5). For health learning to have taken place, there must be a positive change in behavior.

Comprehensive Health Education

Health education works. Hundreds of studies have evaluated health education and concluded that it is effective in reducing the number of teenage pregnancies, decreasing smoking rates among young people, and preventing the adoption of many high-risk behaviors (Summerfield, 1992).

A sequential comprehensive program rather than sporadic health lectures serves best to introduce healthful lifestyle habits; therefore, we should seek to offer comprehensive health education in our schools. A school health education curriculum is an organized, sequential plan for grades kindergarten through 12 for teaching students and helping them develop life skills that will improve their health, prevent diseases, and reduce health-related risk behaviors (Meeks, Heit, & Page, 2009, p. 20).

Fast Facts

It is not enough to offer health education periodically as issues arise. Health should be taught, as other disciplines, by building concepts and skills in a sequential, organized fashion.

Clinical Snapshot

Jennifer, a school nurse and health teacher, was invited into a fifth-grade class to discuss the dangers of smoking. When she began explaining how cigarette residue interferes with the exchange of air in the alveoli, she realized the students had no knowledge of the anatomy

(*continued*)

(continued)

of the lungs. Had this information been included in earlier lessons, a brief review would have been all that was required for the fifth graders. Students could then better understand how harmful smoking is.

Comprehensive health education in the classroom:

- Addresses the physical, mental, emotional, and social dimensions of health
- Develops health knowledge, attitudes, and skills
- Is tailored to each age level
- Is designed to motivate and assist students to maintain and improve their health and prevent disease

Healthy People 2020 Objectives: Early and Middle Childhood, 4.3:
Increase the proportion of schools that require cumulative instruction in health education that meet the U.S. National Health Education Standards for elementary, middle, and high schools:
Elementary—from 7.5% in 2006 to 11.5%
Middle—from 10.3% in 2006 to 14.3%
High—from 6.5% in 2006 to 10.5%

RISK FACTORS FOR YOUNG PEOPLE

The Centers for Disease Control and Prevention (CDC) has identified six categories of priority health-risk behaviors among youth and young adults:

1. Behaviors that contribute to unintentional injuries and violence (accidents, suicides, etc.)
2. Tobacco use
3. Alcohol and drug use
4. Sexual behaviors that contribute to unintended pregnancy and sexually transmitted infections
5. Unhealthful dietary behaviors
6. Physical inactivity

The Youth Risk Behavior Surveillance System

The Youth Risk Behavior Surveillance System (YRBSS) was developed in 1990 to monitor health behaviors that contribute markedly to the leading causes of death, disability, and social problems among youth and adults in the United States. In addition, every 2 years the YRBSS monitors the prevalence of obesity and asthma and other health-related behaviors plus sexual identity and sex of sexual contacts.

From 1991 to 2017, the YRBSS has collected data from more than 4.4 million high school students in more than 1,900 separate surveys. Thirty-nine states are represented in this last report.

Specifically, the YRBSS is designed to:

- Determine the prevalence of certain health behaviors.
- Assess whether health behaviors increase, decrease, or stay the same over time.
- Examine the co-occurrence of health behaviors.
- Provide comparable national, state, territorial, tribal, and local data.
- Provide comparable data among subpopulations of youth.
- Monitor progress toward achieving the *Healthy People* objectives and other program indicators.

Results from the *2017 National Youth Risk Behavior Surveillance Report* indicate that many high school students engage in behaviors that increase their likelihood for the leading causes of death among persons age 10 to 24 years in the United States. The following information summarizes key elements from the 2016–2017 survey. During the 30 days prior to the survey, students reported that:

- 39.2% drove a car while they had texted or emailed
- 29.0% reported current alcohol use
- 19.8% reported current marijuana use
- 14% had taken prescription pain medicine without a doctor's prescription
- 19% had been bullied on school property
- 7.4% had attempted suicide (within the year)
- 8.8% smoked cigarettes
- 43% played video or computer games 3 or more hours per day not related to school work
- 15% had not been physically active for at least 60 minutes per day and were overweight
- 32% of students felt sad or hopeless
- 40% of students were actively having sex (CDC, 2017)

THE NATIONAL HEALTH EDUCATION STANDARDS

To address the preceding concerns, national standards were developed to help states and local districts meet the needs of students in all grade levels from prekindergarten through grade 12. These standards provide health educators with a framework for teachers, administrators, and policy makers in designing or selecting curricula, allocating instructional resources, and assessing student achievement and progress. Importantly, the standards provide students, families, and communities with concrete expectations for health education reflecting the blueprint for local district curriculum development, instruction, and assessment based on the latest research data.

The National Health Education Standards (NHES) are written with expectations for what students should know and be able to do by grades 2, 5, 8, and 12 to promote personal, family, and community health.

Fast Facts

The NHES are written to be deliberately vague, allowing teachers to adapt them to the needs of their individual classes and students.

Clinical Snapshot

Jennifer has just completed screenings in height and weight and calculating body mass indices for students. She notes that 30% of the eighth-grade class is obese. Before developing her lessons, she must identify the common cause and direct her lessons accordingly. Her focus should be on current diet and exercise habits and the long-term effects on health.

In 2006, the Joint Committee on Health Education Standards established the following guidelines for health education:

- Specify what students should know.
- Specify what students should be able to do.
- Knowledge and skills involved are essential to the development of health literacy.
- Skills include communication, reasoning, and investigating.

The NHES include eight standards, described in Table 7.1.

Table 7.1

National Health Education Standards (NHES)

Standard 1	Students will comprehend concepts related to health promotion and disease prevention to enhance health.
Standard 2	Students will analyze the influence of family, peers, culture, media, technology, and other factors on health behaviors.
Standard 3	Students will demonstrate the ability to access valid information and products and services to enhance health.
Standard 4	Students will demonstrate the ability to use interpersonal communication skills to enhance health and avoid or reduce health risks.
Standard 5	Students will demonstrate the ability to use decision-making skills to enhance health.
Standard 6	Students will demonstrate the ability to use goal-setting skills to enhance health.
Standard 7	Students will demonstrate the ability to practice health-enhancing behaviors and avoid or reduce risks.
Standard 8	Students will demonstrate the ability to advocate for personal, family, and community health.

Source: Centers for Disease Control and Prevention. (2017). *Health Insurance Coverage.* Retrieved from https://www.cdc.gov/nchs/fastats/health-insurance.htm

Needs Assessment

Using these national standards as a guide, states and local districts work to address the specific needs of their students and develop further core standards to reference when planning health curricula. From these curricula, the units of instruction are developed, and specific lesson plans are designed.

State Curriculum Content Standards

There are also state curriculum content standards for all disciplines, including health and physical education. These standards are revised at least every 5 years. They provide consistency throughout each state; help improve student learning; form the foundation for assessment, curriculum development, and instruction; and serve as a guide for writing lesson plans.

As an example of these standards, the New Jersey Student Learning Standards for Health are as follows:

- All students will acquire health promotion concepts and skills to support a healthy, active lifestyle.

- All students will develop and use personal and interpersonal skills to support a healthy, active lifestyle.
- All students will acquire knowledge about alcohol, tobacco, other drugs, and medicines and apply these concepts to support a healthy, active lifestyle.
- All students will acquire knowledge about the physical, emotional, and social aspects of human relationships and sexuality and apply these concepts to support a healthy, active lifestyle. (New Jersey Department of Education, 2014)

HEALTH CURRICULUM CONTENT AREAS

School health education programs should be based on local needs—the health behaviors and problems within the school population. Most health professionals would agree that there are 10 general areas to address:

1. Community health
2. Mental consumer health
3. Environmental health
4. Personal health and fitness
5. Family life education
6. Nutrition and healthy eating
7. Disease prevention and control
8. Safety and injury prevention
9. Prevention of substance use and abuse (alcohol, tobacco, drugs)
10. Growth and development

Fast Facts

As you develop your units and lessons, remember that learning will not take place unless the topic is relevant to the needs of the learner. Know your students, and plan accordingly.

Clinical Snapshot

School nurse Jennifer spent hours developing a comprehensive unit on the different food groups for her 10th-grade classes. She is disheartened when students show no interest and were are rude and inattentive. In hindsight, Jennifer realized that this is a boring, repetitive topic for the age group. More relevant topics for high school students would be eating disorders or fad diets.

Health Literacy

An important concept underlying health education is health literacy. This includes having a sound knowledge base so that when students complete their school health education, they can go forward capable of making sound health decisions in their lives. The goal is for every student to think critically, have good communication skills, and be contributing members of society.

TEACHING HEALTH

Steps for Teaching Health

- Identify general health-risk factors of the population as a whole.
- Reference the national and state standards.
- Consider the topics listed for that month by the National Health Observances given in Appendix D.
- Assess your students' needs.
- Develop the curriculum with assistance from colleagues and the administration. Have the curriculum approved by the principal, and present it at an open board meeting where parents can have input.
- Plan the unit of instruction to cover each content area.
- Develop the lesson plan in a way that is specific to the needs of your students.
- Implement the lesson plan.
- Evaluate the lesson plan, and revise it as often as needed to accommodate the changing needs of students.
- Keep parents informed, especially when teaching issues that are controversial or involve sexuality.

In-Service Education for Staff Members

According to state and district policy, teachers and other school staff members must receive instruction on a number of health topics on a yearly or biennial basis. This provides an excellent opportunity for school nurses to demonstrate their teaching skills and establish themselves as health educators.

Procedure for Providing In-Service Education for Staff Members

- Identify topics in your policy and procedure book for which education is required (child abuse, blood-borne pathogens, suicide, anaphylaxis, safety, etc.).

- Write a topic agenda, and have it approved by the school administration.
- Arrange an appropriate time and place for in-service education.
- Develop and deliver a PowerPoint or Webex presentation.
- Have the staff complete an evaluation of your program.
- Award in-service credit if it is given in your district.
- Investigate appropriate online courses of the relevant topics that may be available to teachers.

Role of School Nurses in Health Education

- Be a role model for healthful habits.
- Make resources available to teachers and students.
- Help plan the health curriculum.
- Teach one-on-one, to small groups, or in the classroom.
- Serve as a health consultant to students and colleagues.
- Stay current on health issues.
- Do not allow yourself to become so overwhelmed with procedural tasks and first aid that you have no time to teach, in and out of the classroom.
- Plan additional staff in-service education as issues arise.

OBSTACLES TO CLASSROOM HEALTH TEACHING

Perceived Poor Classroom Management Skills

The most logical approach is to seek assistance from the experienced master teachers in your school or district. Observe them teaching, seek and follow suggestions, and then have them critique your lessons.

Lack of Time to Prepare and Implement Lessons

If you have a teaching schedule or the same contract as your colleagues, you are entitled to preparation time in your schedule. Speak to your administrator or, if necessary, your union representative.

Concern Over Handling Sensitive Issues

Know your curriculum. If it has been board approved and parents have been notified of the content, you may answer questions and deal with sensitive issues in an age-appropriate manner. Notify parents when sensitive sexual topics are planned, and allow them the opportunity to review the lesson content and, if they wish, exclude their children. If a topic repeatedly surfaces with students and it is not part of the curriculum, recommend it be included.

Frustrations With Constant Interruptions or Lack of Health Office Coverage

Clarify with the school administration who will make student assessments, and decide whether to interrupt your class when you are teaching. Define to that person what constitutes a *true* emergency, and give specific instructions about how non-urgent problems are to be handled until you finish teaching and return to the health office.

Low Priority Given to Health Education Compared With Other Disciplines

Students are given standardized tests for math, reading, science, and other content areas. These scores are made public, and schools tend to focus time and energy on raising their students' scores so that they are seen in a favorable light by parents and other districts. Health education is seldom measured with a standardized test that is made public.

School nurses need to remind all involved of the importance of health education and the need for students to be *well enough to learn*. The true test of this goal is students' ability to make good lifestyle choices. This is impossible to measure in the short term.

Fast Facts

Take it upon yourself to initiate opportunities to demonstrate your teaching skills. You are a competent nurse *and* teacher. Sometimes you need to escape from your office to see the bigger picture.

Clinical Snapshot

School nurse Jennifer hates lunchtime recess. There usually is standing room only in the school health office because of numerous playground injuries. Frustrated, she decides to go outside and observe what is going on. She notes that supervision is inadequate and some playground practices are unsafe. Jennifer speaks with the principal and physical education teacher and organizes a safety in-service program on playground use for the staff and lunch aides. Children playing recklessly are made to sit for a designated time. Fewer injuries now occur, and Jennifer has more time to focus on the unavoidable injuries.

References

Centers for Disease Control and Prevention. (2017). *Health Insurance Coverage.* Retrieved from https://www.cdc.gov/nchs/fastats/health-insurance.htm

Gilbert, G. (2000). *Health education: Creating strategies for school and community health.* Sudbury, MA: Jones and Bartlett.

Meeks, L., Heit, P., & Page, R. (2009). *Comprehensive school health education: Totally awesome strategies for teaching health* (6th ed., pp. 4–24). New York, NY: McGraw-Hill.

New Jersey Department of Education. (2014). *School health services guidelines* (pp. 1–141). Trenton, NJ: Author. Retrieved from http://www.state.nj.us/education/students/safety/health/services

Summerfield, L. (1992). *Comprehensive school health education.* ERIC Digest. Ten topic areas to be included in any comprehensive school health program. Retrieved from http://www.ericdigests.org/1992-1/health.htm

III

Professional Issues in School Nursing Practice

8

Documentation in School Nursing Practice

"If it was not documented, it was not done." These might have been among the first words heard when you started your nursing studies. Today the words remain true and carry even greater significance in school health. Remember, a school nurse works alone. If you do not document appropriately, no one else will.

It is no secret that we are living in litigious times. Legal actions against school boards of education are far too common, and the great majority of these actions are centered on the delivery of healthcare. What you do for children is certainly important; however, how you document your actions is just as important. You must always be able to provide written evidence that you acted correctly.

In this chapter, you will learn:

1. Concerns about documentation
2. Information required for students' individual health folders
3. Assessment information needed for daily log entries
4. How to maintain emergency health cards
5. How to complete some administrative reports required in your state and district

DOCUMENTATION CONCERNS

School nurses face decisions every day regarding health information: how much should be written in files, where they should be stored, and who should be permitted to see these files. Often, unauthorized personnel have access to private data.

Recordkeeping tasks are endless and time-consuming. They keep school nurses from spending valuable time directly with their students. We grudgingly do it, and far too frequently, we omit valuable information. Each school district has some variation as to the types of forms used for documentation, but a number of documents are required by all districts.

INDIVIDUAL HEALTH FOLDERS

Every student must have his or her own electronic or hard copy health folder, containing, at a minimum, the following documents:

- A permanent, cumulative health form that includes:
  - The student's birth date
  - The parents' names, address(es), and phone numbers
  - Screening data
  - A record of immunizations
  - Growth and development information
  - Disease history
  - Blood pressure
  - Tuberculosis testing results
  - Lead testing results
  - Dental examination data
  - A nurses' notes section containing the date of enrollment, any transfers, and any further significant health information
- Health information taken from initial registration
- Previous school health records
- An individual student log sheet
- An immunization record
- An individual medication record
- Referrals and follow-ups
- Copies of accident or incident reports
- Any correspondence from parents, physicians, teachers, and so on
- A report of physical examinations
- Notes about any exclusions from physical education classes or school
- Your personal notes, which are not included on the permanent record

Fast Facts

An individual health folder is a legal document. All entries should be made in ink, with the exception of the student's address and phone numbers. Errors should be bracketed and initialed. Do not erase or white out anything that has been written.

Clinical Snapshot

Adriana, the certified school nurse, is paid a stipend to come to school in early August. She personally reviews incoming students' health records. Parents must sign consents for her to receive the information. Adriana insists on this background information from sending districts. Sometimes, her forms are more inclusive than theirs, and further information is needed. Preparing in August gives her time to review information and, with parental written consent, share on a need-to-know basis with staff, before the children enter school in September.

Role of School Nurses in Documentation in Individual Health Folders

- Gather and carefully review all available medical information for the incoming student. Note any restrictions, major illnesses, operations, and so on. If the student is transferring into your school, send for the permanent health record from the previous school, note when the student was admitted to your school in the nurses' notes section, and continue adding information as needed.
- List all information deficiencies, and notify parents of these, along with a deadline for any examination, referral, or immunization required.
- Follow up on all information deficiencies and referrals. Inform the administration of those who are noncompliant.
- If this is the first school for the student or if the health records are unobtainable, note your efforts to obtain the records, the dates of those efforts, and any administration support in getting records. Start a new cumulative, permanent health card.
- Include all information provided to you in the folder.
- Obtain written permission from the parent(s) to share confidential health information with teachers and other personnel whom you deem appropriate.
- Regardless of whether documentation is done electronically or in hard copy form, make sure the information is kept secure. Folders should be stored in a locked file cabinet, and your password for

electronic data should not be shared. Forward information to a sending school only when written parental permission has been obtained and it is permitted by your district policy. Always use discretion.

- When a student transfers out of your district, keep a copy of the permanent health record for your files.
- Maintain student records for the time designated by your district, usually until the student is 21 years old.
- Alphabetically arrange all files according to class or grade level.
- Keep copies of permanent health forms for all students placed out of the district.
- In some districts all school documents are now computerized. The same rules for privacy apply.

Fast Facts

Assembling, reviewing, and entering all this information into a permanent record can be very time-consuming. When a district does not allocate money for summer work, the task is especially frustrating. You will want to have as much done as possible before students start classes yet resent spending your personal time.

Clinical Snapshot

School nurse Adriana completes as much of her charting as possible before the school year ends. As documents arrive, she starts the students' folders and continuously updates. This way, as much as possible is done in advance.

DAILY LOGS

In addition to the cumulative health record, the school nurse must document all student visits to the health office. Ideally, entries should be made immediately. However, the health office is a busy place, and this is often not possible. The following procedure may help you keep track of numerous visits.

Role of School Nurses in Maintaining Daily Logs

- Use a notebook, clipboard, or laptop on which students write their names and times of arrival. Young children should bring passes from their teachers that include the date, time, child's name, and

teacher observations. These notes are available for all to see, so they should contain no further information. Keep these notes and log pages for each student until he or she has graduated or reaches 21 years of age so you can reference them if necessary in a legal action.
- Assess each student using the nursing process: assess, diagnose, plan, implement, and evaluate. Check vital signs, note skin color and body language, and so on.
- Take a history. Ask relevant questions: *Were you sick this morning? What were you doing in class before coming to my office?*
- Speak with a parent or teacher if necessary.
- At this point, do one of three things:
  - Allow the student to rest, and continue to observe him or her.
  - Send the student back to class.
  - Excuse the student from school.
- Check on the student's status later in the day.
- Document your actions on the student's individual log sheet or software standardized form. Include *all* relevant data, conversations, follow-up efforts, and outcome.
- If the incident or illness warrants further clarification, complete an incident report, and file it according to district policy.
- Protect all students' privacy. Do not make their complaints known to others in your office. Keep records in their folders and the folders in the locked file cabinet or under your password in whatever software program you are using.

EMERGENCY HEALTH CARDS/FORMS

Every student and staff member must have annually updated emergency information. Keep emergency information in an accessible but secure location. Save the previous year's data to verify information.

Information Needed on an Emergency Health Card

- Individual's name, address, and home phone number
- Parents' names and addresses if different from the student's
- Parents' email addresses, work, and cell phone numbers
- Several reliable contact people whom you can call if parents are unavailable
- Contact information of staff members' families or friends
- One parent's or guardian's signature
- Name of the legal custodian(s)
- Physician's name and phone number

The emergency health card can also be used to update health information. Add the following question:

Is there any new information regarding your child's health status?
No______Yes______Comment:________________________________.

You may also ask parents to initial a box if they *do not* wish to have health information shared with relevant staff members. This gives you the needed consent in writing.

Include a reminder about the school's medication policy. Add district requirements for returning to school after an illness and the school exclusion policy.

When dealing with an ill child who must be excluded, keep in mind the following:

- Do not allow anyone who is not named on the card to pick up a student unless the parent gives explicit permission. The student should be able to identify that person and appear comfortable with him or her.
- Do not permit a student to leave with anyone he or she does not recognize or whose behavior is inappropriate.
- Always call a parent first regarding illnesses and accidents.
- Do not discuss a student's health problem with anyone who answers the phone at the parent's home or work number.

Role of School Nurses in Keeping Emergency Health Cards

- Be certain that every child and staff member has an annually updated card.
- Make sure cards are all completed accurately and signed by parents or guardians.
- Include a card in the admission packet for newly enrolled students.
- Store information in a secure area.

Fast Facts

Coordinate with nursing colleagues on the keeping and filing of reports. Explore new technology to simplify recordkeeping.

Clinical Snapshot

Adriana is one of several nurses in the district. She needs to collaborate with her district colleagues to unify the approach to paperwork. It will be easier for any substitutes and save time and money in the long run.

ADMINISTRATIVE REPORTS

The school nurse is responsible for a number of reports throughout the school year. Not all reports are required by every school, district, or state. Check with your administration to see what is relevant for you and the date on which any reports are due. Some of the more commonly requested reports are described in the following sections.

Daily, Weekly, Monthly, and Annual Reports

These reports are made upon a request and help justify how you are spending your time. Prepare a checklist of the number of health office visits, exclusions, medications given, phone conferences, screenings performed, deficiency notices sent out, classes taught, and so on. This is an excellent way to communicate with your administrator and keep a record of statistics.

Child Study Team

Every child who is evaluated by the child study team should have input from the school nurse. Prepare a report that includes a summary of the last physical examination and any health problem that could interfere with learning. Attend the meeting to discuss your findings, especially if there are significant medical issues.

504 Accommodations

Students with 504 Accommodation Plans have difficulty with one or more activities of daily living. There are children who require accommodations during the school day so that maximum learning can take place. Be aware of these children, know the extent of the required accommodations, and ensure that the accommodations are implemented.

Tuberculosis Report

Most states require some type of report so they can follow up on the incidence of tuberculosis. This is how they evaluate the need for testing in particular areas. Standardized forms asking for the number of students and staff tested and the results are usually sent by the state and must be completed by the school nurse.

Immunization Status Report

Once you have completed checking all your students' immunizations, you must file an annual report with the state. It includes information on the number of students with provisional admission as well as those with medical, philosophical, and religious exemptions.

Nursing Service Plan

Some states require an annual quality assurance report. Part of this report asks school nurses to identify those students needing specialized nursing care. It is designed to make sure students with medical needs are cared for adequately.

Role of School Nurses in Filing Administrative Reports

- Know what—and when—reports are due for your district.
- Keep careful records so retrieving the information will be easy.
- Use this information to support your need for more nursing assistance.

Accident or Incident Reports

An accident or incident report is a written statement by an eyewitness, which is obtained and provided as part of the legal record as close to the time of the event as possible. It is part of the overall risk management program of any institution's policy, including school district policy. Accident or incident reports are generally used post incident to review and evaluate nursing care; to monitor equipment, the grounds, and buildings for unsafe conditions; and to document events in anticipation of insurance claims (Schwab & Gelfman, 2001).

The person who actually witnesses an incident should provide the firsthand information. If no adult observed an incident firsthand, the nurse should document in the form, for example, "Mrs. Smith stated that Robert fell, hitting his head."

Role of School Nurses in Reporting Accidents or Incidents

- Keep in mind the importance of prevention. The school nurse's first task is to anticipate accidents as much as possible. Be involved in risk management and assessment in the building and on the playground.
- Keep the administration informed of potential problems, as well as immediately following an incident.
- Periodically call the local police department to see if injuries have occurred after hours on playground equipment or the school grounds. If repeated accidents occur on the same equipment, it should be evaluated for defects.

- Keep detailed records and reports of all potentially libelous incidents. Any situation that is out of the ordinary should be noted.
- Include only factual information relevant to an incident.
- In addition to an accident report, you must still enter the information on the student's personal log sheet as you would for any health office visit.

Reference

Schwab, N., & Gelfman, M. (Eds.). (2001). *Legal issues in school health services: A resource for school administrators, school attorneys and school nurses* (pp. 499–500). North Branch, MN: Sunrise River Press.

9

Legal Considerations in School Nursing Practice

The surest way to get hired for a school nurse position is to stress the fact that you will carefully follow school policies and procedures to keep your district within the law. The surest way not to get hired is to be totally naive about the very real possibility that you could be involved in a lawsuit. Unfortunately, schools are always under scrutiny, and the school nurse is frequently at the forefront of a pending lawsuit.

Today's school is a complex legal environment. You will learn quickly that nothing is more important to a board of education than feeling totally comfortable knowing that the school nurse is aware of the basic legal framework governing schools and will be protectively proactive for the district and himself or herself.

In this chapter, you will learn:

1. The three levels of laws
2. Elements of the different classifications of laws
3. Distinctions among liability, negligence, and malpractice
4. Major areas of potential liability
5. Strategies to avoid lawsuits

LEVELS OF LAWS

Laws are written and enacted at three levels: federal, state, and local.

Federal Laws

In 1791, the Tenth Amendment of the U.S. Constitution gave authority to the individual states in educational matters. Federal laws and policies usually defer to state and local governments, provided that they do not violate any constitutional rights.

These laws apply to everyone in the United States. Federal laws deal with immigration, social security, federal criminal laws, tax fraud, and counterfeiting.

The federal government collaborates with state and local school districts to improve public education. The federal government may fund educational programs contingent on the implementation of specific policies.

State Laws

The state has the authority to act in the interest of protecting the citizens of that state. State laws would deal with divorces, welfare, wills, inheritance, real estate, business contracts, personal injury, medical malpractice, and workman's compensation.

The state also has significant power to determine minimum school attendance requirements, curricula, and educational requirements. In recognition of the Tenth Amendment, states have had full and complete jurisdiction in educational matters and can delegate certain power to local school districts.

Local Laws

Local laws deal only with matters relevant to a particular municipality. These laws deal with rents, zoning, health issues, local safety issues, and so on.

All states have district school boards of education whose members are either appointed by local government officials or elected by popular vote. These boards of education can determine the specific content of curricula, raise funds, and hire personnel. The local district determines the instructional methods and materials to be used to best meet their students' needs.

CLASSIFICATIONS OF LAWS

There are three basic classifications of laws in the United States: criminal, civil, and administrative. School nurses need to know the parameters of each classification.

Criminal Laws

These are statutes enacted to maintain order and protect society as a whole. There are, for example, laws against the crimes of theft, illegal drug use, libel, slander, medical malpractice, practicing without a license, failing to report child abuse, tampering with official records, and kidnapping.

Civil Laws

These laws protect the rights of the individual. Enforcement of civil laws often involves an attempt to find a peaceable resolution through compensation or by stopping the actionable practice. The Family Educational Rights and Privacy Act (FERPA) of 1974 and the Health Insurance Portability and Accountability Act (HIPAA) of 1996 are examples of civil laws.

Family Educational Rights and Privacy Act

FERPA is a federal law that protects the privacy of student educational records. It applies to all schools that receive funds under an applicable program of the U.S. Department of Education. The act contains the following provisions:

- Parents have the right to access their children's educational records.
- All school records are considered educational.
- Personally identifiable student information contained in health records must be protected.
- Sensitive records, such as those concerning child abuse, and psychological and counseling information, should be kept separate and secure.
- Access is limited to those with a "legitimate educational interest."
- Student files kept on computers must have safeguards in place to ensure the same level of security.
- Parental consent is required before records can be transferred to a new school.

Health Insurance Portability and Accountability Act

HIPAA was written to address the concern of maintaining the confidentiality of health records transmitted electronically. Among its key provisions are the following:

- The primary goal is to make it easier for people to retain health insurance, protect confidentiality, and help control administrative costs in healthcare.

- There are two separate sections: Title I deals with portability, allowing individuals to carry health insurance from one job to another. Title II deals with administrative simplification by setting standards for receiving, transmitting, and maintaining healthcare information and ensuring privacy.
- Compliance is focused on healthcare providers or agencies that bill the individual.
- HIPAA provides that patients have a right to receive notice of the privacy practices of the provider.
- It was not intended to interfere with the sharing of necessary health information between the school and healthcare providers. Schools and physicians are considered "covered entities," and information can be shared on a need-to-know basis. Written permission from the parent is required.

Administrative Laws

Criminal and civil laws determine what can or cannot be done in particular situations. Administrative laws determine who will interpret, enforce, and regulate laws. Agencies such as state boards of nursing are given the responsibility of handling such statutory laws pertaining to nursing. They have the authority to revoke nurses' licenses when nurses have not met the standards of care set forth by the state's nurse practice act (Selekman, 2006, p. 298).

LIABILITY, NEGLIGENCE, AND MALPRACTICE

To be *liable* for something is to be responsible for one's own conduct. In our schools today, two principles should guide our actions: *reasonableness* and *in loco parentis*. Nurses and teachers are expected to act in a *reasonable* fashion. *In loco parentis* means "in place of the parent." This identifies the protective relationship of nurses and teachers to students. It justifies their ability and responsibility to take care of students' needs.

A nurse is considered *negligent* if he or she fails to act in a manner in which another nurse in a similar situation would have acted and his or her performance falls below a reasonable *standard of care*. For the school nurse, the degree of care that another prudent school nurse under the same set of circumstances would have rendered indicates whether an action was negligent.

Malpractice is negligence by a professional person, such as a physician or nurse.

Fast Facts

School districts carry the necessary malpractice insurance to cover employees. School nurses are included in this coverage. However, many nurses carry their own individual malpractice insurance because of the additional benefits provided, which cover them whether or not they are working in the school.

Clinical Snapshot

School nurse Beverly has been employed by the same district for more than 10 years. She also works per diem at the local community hospital. Both school and hospital cover her while she is employed; however, Beverly also carries a separate policy that covers her individually for all other nursing services and provides added protection should she be sued in any capacity.

LEGAL ISSUES AND THE COORDINATED SCHOOL HEALTH PROGRAM

As mentioned in Chapter 1, Bed Baths to Band-Aids: What the School Nurse Really Does, the Coordinated School Health Program includes eight components that cover all areas of student and staff needs. These areas are used as a reference point by Collins, Goodman, and Moulton (2008) in their Centers for Disease Control and Prevention review of what the laws require of schools. A summary of some potential liability issues are identified for each component, along with suggested strategies that school nurses can use to avoid legal encounters.

Health Education

- *Issue:* Health lessons on sensitive topics such as sexuality, emotional health, and substance abuse.
- *Strategies:* Work within your approved health curriculum. Never ask personal questions. Make sure you receive proper training. Send home written notices of topics to be covered. Allow parents the opportunity to review the curriculum and exclude their child.

Physical Education and Activity

Issues: Equal opportunity to participate in sports for both sexes, adaptive physical education, individualized education plans (IEPs) and individualized healthcare plans (IHPs), sports injuries, protective gear, proper supervision, staff training in cardiopulmonary resuscitation (CPR) and use of *automated external defibrillators* (AED), and gym participation exemptions.

Strategies: Check that sport activities are offered for girls. Review IEPs and IHPs to make sure students with special needs receive adaptive physical education if included in their IEP. See that helmets, safety glasses, and so on are available and worn. Look into the student–teacher ratio of physical education classes. Offer CPR/AED classes to physical education teachers and any other staff member who requests certification.

Exemptions and restrictions must be clarified by a physician and honored by physical education teachers. Check dates and types of restrictions. Use caution in allowing students to return to full activity. Keep physical education teachers informed of students with restrictions and of when they are cleared to return to class.

Fast Facts

Even if a student has been cleared for return to full participation in physical education, consider the anticipated activity before allowing the student to return.

Clinical Snapshot

Lisa, age 6, was casted for 6 weeks following a fracture in her right wrist. She presents a note from her orthopedist, stating that she is cleared to return to gym and allowed to participate in all activities. School nurse Beverly is aware that Lisa's physical education class will be doing exercises using the monkey bars. She can suggest that Lisa avoid this specific activity for a few more weeks, knowing it will place tremendous strain on her newly healed wrist.

Health Services

- *Issues:* First aid, emergency care, medications, screenings, routine and sports assessments, privacy, child abuse, communicable diseases, and students with special needs.
- *Strategies:* Have annually updated, signed standing orders, IEPs, and emergency care plans. Maintain current CPR/AED certifications. Carefully note health issues, especially heart defects, chronic conditions, seizure disorders, and so on. Include actions

to be taken for a classroom emergency. Perform and accurately document first aid and medication administration according to school policy and procedures. Administer only medications that must be given in school. Attend and be vocal at child study team meetings. Follow up on all screening referrals. Report suspicion of child abuse to the proper agency. Know and report rare infectious diseases as required by local policy. Report high levels of communicable diseases to county and state authorities.

Fast Facts

If a child has a known cardiac condition for which he or she is being followed by a cardiologist, request that the cardiologist, not the pediatrician, clear him or her for participation in physical education.

Clinical Snapshot

School nurse Beverly enrolls a new student from an Asian country. The physical examination form has been signed by a local pediatrician and returned, indicating that the student is cleared for all activity. However, in reviewing a previous physical exam record from the student's country of origin, Beverly sees a notation indicating that he had a period of apnea at 18 months. Beverly knows that the pediatrician is not fluent in the student's first language and questions whether this information was shared during the most recent examination. Beverly suggests an interpreter return with the parents and sends a copy of the previous physical examination. If Beverly is not satisfied that the cardiac condition is addressed properly, she can discuss the student with the school physician before permitting the child to participate in physical education.

Nutrition Services

- *Issues:* Anaphylaxis, nutritious lunch offerings, cleanliness and behavior in the lunchroom, and rights of children with food allergies
- *Strategies:* Educate lunchroom staff about signs and symptoms of anaphylaxis. Keep an epinephrine auto-injector available. Check that dietary regulations are followed. Form a committee of parents of children with food allergies. Consider their input on how to protect their children while allowing socialization. Insist on adequate lunchroom supervision. Hang a poster demonstrating the Heimlich maneuver in the lunchroom, and annually train the lunchroom aides in how to administer it.

Mental Health and Social Services

- *Issues:* Child neglect and abuse, mental health problems (e.g., depression, suicide).
- *Strategies:* If needed, see that counseling services are provided for students or staff. Know your students and your limitations. Immediately report any suspicions of child abuse, depression, and suicidal thoughts expressed by students. Do not try to treat or counsel these students. Work with other professionals in the district to get the appropriate professional help.

Healthful and Safe School Environment

- *Issues:* Indoor air quality, noise, physical security of the building, heating, air conditioning, asbestos, radon, lead contamination in drinking water, injuries caused by unsafe equipment, fire drills, maintenance of fire extinguishers and detectors, school bus safety, pedestrian safety, violence, locker searches, substance abuse, alcohol use, inappropriate student–staff relationships, and school disasters.
- *Strategies:* Refer complaints of environmental issues immediately, and follow up. Question whether proper inspections have been made for drinking fountains, asbestos, playground equipment safety, and so on. Look into school bus safety, seat belt availability, and bus driver complaints and supervision. Insist on a no-bullying, no-violence district policy. Report and document all violent behavior and bullying incidents. Do not become involved in any search of a student for drugs or weapons, whether the student is dressed or undressed.

Health Promotion for Staff

- *Issues:* Physical exams, privacy, 504 accommodations.
- *Strategies:* Cooperate with the administration in obtaining physical examinations of employees. Store files in the most secure location. Administer and follow up on tuberculosis testing. Provide recommendations for 504 accommodations for staff as needed. Remain a health resource for staff. Remain discreet about staff personal issues.

Parent/Family and Community Involvement

- *Issues:* Policy and decision-making dilemmas, parental consent for certain services, and privacy concerns.

- *Strategies:* Encourage partnerships with parent and community groups. Solicit parent involvement as much as possible. Communicate frequently with parents via newsletters, meetings, and office visits. Remain accessible.

Fast Facts

You may also have legal counsel provided through your teacher's union. Explore your possible sources before a need arises.

Clinical Snapshot

Beverly is employed as a school nurse under a teacher's contract and has union dues deducted annually from her pay. She checks with her union leader and learns that she is entitled to 30 minutes of legal advice in any area she needs—home purchase, divorce, writing a will—in addition to school issues.

Role of School Nurses in School Law

- Know and remain current on the laws relevant to your district, state, and country.
- Seek legal advice as needed.
- Remain flexible so you can adapt to religious and ethnic diversities.
- Document and save all correspondence from parents, colleagues, students, outside agencies, and so on.
- Maintain professionalism.
- Notify appropriate people, in writing, of legal concerns.
- Practice preventive strategies to avoid legal problems.

References

Collins, J., Goodman, R., & Moulton, A. (2008). A CDC review of school laws and policies concerning child and adolescent health. *Journal of School Health, 78*(2), 69–119. doi:10.1111/j.1746-1561.2007.00272_1.

Selekman, J. (Ed.). (2006). *School nursing: A comprehensive text*. Philadelphia: F.A. Davis.

10

High-Risk Areas in School Nursing Practice

Every day, the school nurse must decide how best to handle certain situations. The school nurse has standing orders for routine care and for individualized health and emergency care plans that address students with specific needs. However, for people on the front lines of the healthcare delivery system, many situations can arise that have no definitive right or wrong resolution. States, school districts, and professional ethics may be in conflict. Families and communities differ, as resources, values, and expectations are unique to every person and vary by community. What is acceptable in one school, community, or state may not be acceptable in another.

In this chapter, you will learn:

1. The reasons school nurses are at a high risk for liability
2. How to balance the responsibilities of the nursing profession and school policies
3. Areas of conflict in school nursing practice

HIGH-RISK ASPECTS OF SCHOOL HEALTH NURSING PRACTICE

Certain aspects of school health practices put school nurses at higher risk for liability than their colleagues in some other settings, including the following:

- Professional isolation
- A wide range of responsibilities
- Conflicts between policies of boards of education and professional standards of care
- Conflicts between education law and health law (Schwab & Gelfman, 2001, p. 77)

Fast Facts

A school setting is quite different from a hospital. In an acute care setting, a nurse is surrounded by other competent health professionals, has access to diagnostic equipment, and is in an acute care mind-set. In contrast, seldom does a school nurse work with another nurse of equal stature, and never is there a physician on site. Available equipment consists of a thermometer, stethoscope, and blood pressure machine. The focus is on prevention rather than intervention.

Clinical Snapshot

School nurse Andrea is summoned from lunch to evaluate Katherine, a 10-year-old student. Katherine went to the principal's office, stating, "*I can't breathe.*" The principal panicked and immediately called for Andrea. When Andrea arrives, she notes that Katherine's color is fine, her air exchange is good, and respirations are easy at 20. Andrea gives her water and allows her to rest. While talking with Katherine, Andrea learns she has been excluded from a circle of girls and is very unhappy. Andrea summons the other girls to talk about the cruel behavior and privately discusses the overreaction with Katherine.

Consider a child who is truly in respiratory distress and is brought to the emergency department. Some time has already lapsed since the first symptom appeared, and numerous people have already seen the patient. An assessment has been made, and it was determined that immediate care was needed at a hospital facility.

The hospital staff then addresses these needs and intervenes to choose the level of care required. The pulse-oxygen level is checked immediately, and oxygen can be started. An IV infusion with appropriate medication, a nebulizer, or both will be administered. Blood will be drawn and sent out stat. All personnel are prepared to perform cardiopulmonary resuscitation if needed.

In contrast, in the school setting, the nurse must assess alone with limited diagnostic tools. He or she might call for an ambulance without being certain that a student is indeed in distress. Perhaps this is a student who frequently seeks out the school nurse. Did an embarrassing incident trigger a dramatic reaction in the student? Is the distress caused by a reason totally unrelated to illness? Would a drink of water, a puff from an inhaler, or a little downtime and some kind words be all the student needs?

The school nurse has very few minutes to process all of these possibilities. How accurately you make assessments and appropriate decisions, and balance your numerous tasks, will depend largely on the type and years of your nursing experience, educational preparation, and personal, professional, and ethical beliefs.

Fast Facts

Most school nurses have already had some hospital or acute care experience. School experience will come in time, but each situation in the school setting is unique and requires individualized care and attention.

Clinical Snapshot

Mary Beth is one of those students who needs to see you every day. She is a 10th grader with an unstable home life who always appears sad. Today she complains of vague *stomach pains.* School nurse Andrea allows her to stay and tries to engage her in conversation. Her affect is different, and her poor color is noted. When Andrea palpates her abdomen, tenderness is apparent. Playing it safe, Andrea calls home and suggests she be seen immediately by a physician.

Your educational level will depend on what the law requires in the state in which you practice. However, all professionals must continue to learn. If you do not have the skills required for the school setting, you must get them from nursing colleagues, an acute care setting, continuing education, or an academic program in a college or university. Each state has its own board of nursing and nurse practice act defining the scope of practice, but some issues vary across state lines.

The school nurse's job is multifaceted and little understood by other school personnel. While you are attempting to assess a child with respiratory symptoms, other children may continue to arrive for their medications, a diabetic student may need to be tested, and no one else will be available to do these tasks. There are always myriad opportunities for errors to be made. In spite of this overwhelming responsibility, there are teachers and administrators who believe that unless you are teaching 25 students all day, every day, you are not working. A great deal of what school nurses do must be held in confidence; consequently, few people truly know (or care) how you fill your days.

The school nurse stands with one foot in each discipline: nursing and education. As nurses, we must abide by our state's nurse practice act, as the state board of nursing issues our licenses. As teachers, we are employed by the local board of education and obliged to heed federal, state, and district regulations regarding educational matters.

In truth, we serve many masters: several layers of government, our nursing profession, school principals, directors of special services, state boards of nursing, teacher's unions, parents, and so on.

NEGLIGENCE

Negligence cases against school nurses are usually based on allegations that an action taken (or not taken) does not meet the current standards of care. This means that another competent nurse would not have acted in the same way. Some examples of negligence include failure to:

- Keep abreast of current nursing knowledge.
- Document adequately.
- Recognize urgent and emergency situations.
- Follow school district policy.
- Challenge administrative decisions that put students at risk. (Schwab & Gelfman, 2001, p. 77)

SCHOOL NURSE DILEMMAS

The following are theoretical scenarios highlighting some of the dilemmas faced by today's school nurses. As has been mentioned, there are no right or wrong solutions. These scenarios are intended simply to provoke thoughtful discussions.

Issue: Health Office Coverage
Conflict: Nurse practice act versus local board of education
Scenario: A second grader, Emily, is sent to you at 9:55 a.m. and is obviously acutely ill. You are expected to teach a health lesson to her class at 10:00 a.m. You have 5 minutes to assess, call her parent, and get to class.

Discussion Points:

- If you are late to your class, the teacher will not get his or her full preparation time, as granted in his or her (and your) contract. The teacher could file a grievance.
- Was this child sent to school ill, and why did the teacher not send her to you earlier?
- Should you:
  - Bring Emily with you and assess her after class?
  - Take her temperature quickly, call a parent, and have her wait to be picked up in the main office, perhaps excluding a well child or exposing the secretary and others to illness?
  - Stay with her, assess her properly, and allow her to rest on your cot until she feels better and can return to class or until the parent arrives?
  - Make up the health class at a later time in the day or week instead of doing what you had originally planned to do at that time?
  - See if someone else can teach your health class? (Good luck!)

Issue: Clearance to Participate in Sports

Conflict: Private physician versus school physician

Scenario: You note on Luke's assessment record that he has a history of a mild concussion at age 10. He is now a high school senior, and you know that he has had at least two other head injuries during soccer games. His private physician has cleared him to participate in football. You report this to the school physician, who refuses to allow him to participate in football. The principal and Luke's parents are angry with you for "making such a big deal" about his history of head injuries.

Discussion Points:

- Who has ultimate authority in decisions like this?
- Should you have raised the question?
- Is there a school policy to back up the exclusion?
- Is the coach given input?
- Can you legally refuse to sign clearance, along with the school physician?
- How will your decision affect your tenure and your job?
- Are you willing to risk the unrest your decision will cause?

Issue: Child Abuse

Conflict: Ethical beliefs versus local district policy

Scenario: Maria is a 12-year-old special education student who, following a class on puberty, tearfully confides to you that her

19-year-old mentally challenged cousin fondles her when they are alone. Maria likes her cousin and denies having had intercourse or ever being forced to allow him to touch her. She begs you to keep this in confidence and swears she will never be alone with her cousin again. Maria fears that her father will physically harm both her cousin and her if he finds out.

Discussion Points:

- Who should address this situation: the school guidance counselor or administration, the children's protective services agency, or the parents?
- Will outside agency involvement cause upheaval in their close Hispanic family?
- As both parties are special education students involved in consensual acts, is this a reportable issue?
- Should you agree to keep Maria's confidence and privately work with the parents?
- Since the incidents occur off school premises, how much involvement is it appropriate for you to have?

Issue: Immunizations

Conflict: National and state laws versus state health department and local district policy

Scenario: A family has just immigrated to the United States from a war-torn country. They arrive at the school to register their children but have no health records or immunization documentation. You are fairly certain that they are illegal residents.

Discussion Points:

- As all students are entitled to a free and public education, should you find a clinic to provide immunizations and other health services for the family?
- The family does not have a record of any vaccines. Should you exclude them until they can provide evidence of beginning a series of vaccinations?
- Should you stall as long as possible, as you believe that they will probably move anyway?
- Can you share your suspicions of the family's nonresidency status with the administration?

Issue: Do-Not-Resuscitate Order

Conflict: Personal and professional ethics versus parental orders

Scenario: Catherine is a seventh grader in the final stages of cancer. Her parents have refused further treatment and have requested that no heroic measures be offered. Catherine is to attend school as long as possible, and her parents willingly signed a do-not-resuscitate order.

Discussion Points:

- Can you watch a child stop breathing and stand by without attempting to help her?
- Are these parents setting the school up for legal action?
- If you do nothing, will this result in a lawsuit anyway?
- Are the parents justified in refusing further treatment?
- How can you protect this child while she is in school?
- How can you help the teachers and classmates deal with this tragic situation?

Issue: Confidentiality

Conflict: Teachers' need-to-know versus parental rights

Scenario: Eduardo is 11 years old and has a seizure disorder that is well controlled with medication you administer daily at noon. His parents refuse to sign permission for you to share this information with his teachers or anyone else.

Discussion Points:

- How will you prepare Eduardo's teachers for a possible emergency without telling them about his history of seizures?
- Where and how will you document his diagnosis and medication use?
- How will you balance the teachers' need-to-know with the parents' right to privacy?
- Should you share this information with the school physician and the administration?

Issue: Emergency Treatment

Conflict: Nurse practice act versus local district policy

Scenario: Jacob is brought to your office by the physical education teacher with an audible wheeze diaphoretic, and he is clearly struggling to breathe. He has no history of obstructive airway disease. You direct the teacher to call for an ambulance and listen to Jacob's lungs. You clearly hear very poor air exchange and recognize his immediate need for a bronchodilator. You have on hand a nebulizer, tubing, mask, and another student's medication. The paramedics are at least 10 minutes away, and your standing orders do not cover you to medicate in this instance.

Discussion Points:

- Should you try to calm Jacob down, give him water and wait, hoping that his symptoms lessen?
- Are you comfortable enough with your assessment skills to go ahead with the treatment?
- Are you subjecting yourself to a possible lawsuit either way?
- Should you try to call Jacob's physician, and lose valuable time, to get verbal permission to treat him?

Healthy People 2020 Objectives:
Respiratory Diseases, 3.1:
Reduce the emergency department visits for asthma among children and adults aged 5 to 64 years from 57.0% per 10,000 in 2005–2007 to 49.7% per 10,000.

Issue: Administrator Responsibility

Conflict: Administrative authority versus nurse practice act

Scenario: Kevin falls from the top of the monkey bars and hits his head during the lunchtime recess. He is brought to your office, complaining of a headache, and appears to be stunned. You notice that his pupils are not equally reactive to light. You begin to call for an ambulance. The principal admonishes you, telling you that you are overreacting and should call a parent first to carry out his or her wishes.

Discussion Points:

- Should you listen to the principal?
- Should you call a parent and discuss the situation further with the principal?
- Do you have any written procedure for head injuries?

Issue: Searches

Conflict: Privacy rights versus local school district policy

Scenario: You arrive at your high school one morning and are told that you are to assist with a locker search for drugs and weapons. You ask if there is cause for concern and are not given any information.

Discussion Points:

- As the school nurse, should you be part of this process?
- Have students and parents been informed of the search?
- Should you help without additional information?
- If requested, should you search students' bodies for drugs or weapons?

ROLE OF SCHOOL NURSES IN HIGH-RISK AREAS

- Recognize high-risk areas.
- Be proactive, and anticipate dilemmas.
- Seek additional educational preparation as needed. If you have not had acute care experience, get it.
- Stay connected to nursing colleagues and professional organizations.
- Keep careful records; document accurately and appropriately.
- Stay in acute care mode. Be alert for any emergency.

Fast Facts

The school nurse must deal alone with many controversial areas. Seek to gain trust and confidence from parents, administration, and the school board so that they will support your efforts in any situation, regardless of outcome.

Clinical Snapshot

School nurse Andrea has no standing orders to give acetaminophen or ibuprofen. A 16-year-old female student arrives in her office, complaining of dizziness. The student's oral temperature is 103.8°F. Andrea immediately has her lie down; puts cold compresses on her head, axilla, and groin; removes her sneakers; gives a large glass of water; and administers an appropriate dose of liquid ibuprofen. Within a few minutes, the temperature is down, and the student feels better. Andrea calls the student's mom and confesses giving medication without permission. She also informs the principal and school doctor. All are grateful, and Andrea subsequently has ibuprofen added to the list of medications she may give for a temperature above 102°F.

- Remember that the school administrator is not licensed to assess a child, but you are.
- Remain in charge in emergency situations.
- Know district policies and procedures. Challenge those in conflict with your professional beliefs before they become issues

Reference

Schwab, N., & Gelfman, M. (Eds.). (2001). *Legal issues in school health services: A resource for school administrators, school attorneys and school nurses* (pp. 499–500). North Branch, MN: Sunrise River Press.

IV

The Marginalized Child

11

Children With Special Needs

An anecdote from New England goes like this:

> *A group of children is waiting to enter school early one morning. A surprise snowstorm has made the front steps impassable, and the janitor is shoveling the stairs as the children wait.*
>
> *A small boy in a wheelchair says, "Sir, could you please shovel the ramp so I can get in?"*
>
> *Impatiently, the janitor responds, "These kids are waiting to use the stairs. As soon as I get the steps cleared, I will shovel the ramp. You will have to wait."*
>
> *"But," says the little boy, "if you shovel off the ramp, we can all get in." (Lavoie, 2005)*

Children with special needs are now, and forever will be, in the building. Federal laws have made this a reality, and it is the job of school nurses to help them succeed. To do this, we must look closely at who these children with special needs are.

In this chapter, you will learn:

1. Definitions of *impairment, disability, handicap*, and *special needs* and the history of special education in our country
2. The general provisions of, and major differences between, the Americans With Disabilities Act (ADA) and the Individuals

With Disabilities Education Act (IDEA) and how they affect children with special needs
3. How to write appropriate individualized healthcare and emergency health plans
4. How demonstrating knowledge and compassion for children with special needs and their parents is part of the school nurse's role as health counselor

CHILDREN WITH SPECIAL NEEDS

When we hear that a child has "special needs," we might immediately assume that the child has a physical handicap and is confined to a wheelchair. A wheelchair is a visible sign that accommodations must be made for the child. We step aside, hold open the door, and stand ready to assist in any way possible.

The sad truth is that most children with special needs have problems that cannot be seen. A disability may not be readily apparent to casual observers. These children look the same as other children; therefore, they are expected to behave the same.

Impairment

An impairment is a problem with body function or structure. An impairment can be physical, sensory, or developmental in nature.

Disability

A disability is the result of an impairment. A physical impairment would be cerebral palsy. Visual or auditory deficits would be considered sensory impairments. Pervasive developmental disorder is developmental in nature. Disability is thus a complex phenomenon in which impairments interfere with the interaction between features of a person's body and features of the societal norms in which he or she lives (World Health Organization, n.d.). The disability can be:

- Inherited: Genetically transmitted
- Congenital: Obtained during gestation
- Acquired: Through illness or injury
- Of unknown origin

Whether the disability is permanent or transient, mild or severe, or in one or multiple areas, the student will have difficulty behaving and learning in the same way as his or her peers.

Handicap

A child with a handicap has a disadvantage in some way that makes achievement unusually difficult. Academic success can be impeded by hearing or vision loss. A child who is emotionally disturbed will not be able to function to his or her full capacity.

Special Needs

This is an umbrella term that includes children with medical, behavioral, developmental, learning, or mental health issues. These issues cover a wide array of diagnoses.

Fast Facts

Recent years have brought tremendous progress in diagnosing and educating the student with special needs of a physical nature, but we still may not recognize the full potential of the child with mental disabilities.

Clinical Snapshot

Two students in the third grade have special needs. Maria has cerebral palsy and walks with a typical scissor gait. Michael has Asperger's syndrome and is socially compromised. School nurse Emily notices that classmates are overly indulgent in helping Maria navigate about the room but completely intolerant of Michael's behavior. Emily realizes that this is an ideal time and age to speak with and demonstrate acceptance of those with mental special needs. She works with the classroom teacher to educate children in how they can approach, befriend, and accept Michael as a unique member of their class.

The specifics of what caused the special need are well beyond the scope of this book and, in reality, are of little relevance. A person's brain might be wired differently, his or her body may not perform competently, and he or she may or may not look different from others. Regardless of the problem, it cannot be changed. The condition exists, and a child's disability may have an impact on his or her school performance. The school nurse is part of the team whose task is to maximize these students' educational experience, help them avoid complications, and, ideally, enable the student to blend into the school community. Accomplishing this is a significant challenge.

Delegation of Tasks

Today's advances in healthcare and current legislation have enabled children with increasingly complex behavioral and medical needs to be part of the mainstream. It may be necessary for the school nurse to delegate some of the responsibility for their care.

The American Nurses Association (ANA) has defined nursing delegation as the transferring of responsibility for performing a nursing activity to another person while retaining accountability for the outcome (ANA & the National Council of State Boards of Nursing [NCSBN], 2005).

The registered nurse uses critical thinking and professional judgment when following the Five Rights of Delegation, to be sure that the delegation or assignment is:

1. The right task
2. Under the right circumstances
3. To the right person
4. With the right directions and communication
5. Under the right supervision and evaluation (NCSBN)

Delegation should occur on a case-by-case basis within the parameters of the state laws that regulate nursing practice.

Delegation to unlicensed assistive personnel should be considered when a child's medical condition warrants immediate attention, as with anaphylaxis. The school nurse provides the necessary training and supervision. Today most states permit school nurses to train delegates for epinephrine and glucagon administration.

Healthy People 2020 Objectives:
Disability and Health, 14:
Increase the proportion of children and youth with disabilities who spend at least 80% of their time in regular educational programs from 56.8% in 2007–2008 to 73.8%.

HISTORY OF SPECIAL EDUCATION

The history of how society has treated those with special needs is *not* one to be proud of. In the early 1800s, many people were superstitious about those who had mental or physical disabilities. Parents who had the emotional and financial resources kept such children at home and simply managed as best they could. Ashamed of their offspring, parents without resources sometimes abandoned these children and allowed them to die, believing that these "bad" children might be possessed by the devil.

The later 1800s saw the beginnings of institutions for persons with special needs. The objectives were clear. These people were to be given humane treatment yet kept apart from "normal" people. Education was not even a consideration.

Once compulsory school attendance was mandated in the early 1900s, states were forced to recognize the large numbers of students with special needs. Such children could still be excluded, but by gathering together, these children and their parents began to have a voice. That voice grew stronger and soon demanded to be heard by lawmakers.

In 2015–2016, the number of students ages 3 to 21 receiving special education services was 6.7 million, or 13%, of all public school students. Among students receiving special education services, 34% had specific learning disabilities (National Center for Educational Statistics, 2017).

Many more children were not receiving special education services but needed some type of classroom accommodations.

Fast Facts

If you have a self-contained special education class in your building, try to spend time in it. Ask to be included in some of their activities so the children will be comfortable with you. Allow the special education student to do small tasks in the health office: arrange supplies, set up bandages, and so on.

Clinical Snapshot

School nurse Emily suggests that when children are ready to be mainstreamed, they start in her health class. Emily is aware of each child's special needs and is able to deal with him or her appropriately. Depending on the area of need and the class, small group activities can be arranged to provide acceptance and learning opportunities for all.

LEGISLATION

In the early 1970s, public consciousness of people with disabilities was raised. Before that time, there were few educational choices for children with special needs. By 1975, two pieces of federal legislation were in place that had a significant impact on the educational process of special needs students:

- Section 504 of the Rehabilitation Act
- The Education for All Handicapped Children Act

In 1990, those laws were amended and expanded to include even more services for children with special needs. Today, they are known as the ADA, P.L. 101–336, and the IDEA, P.L. 101–476.

Both laws broaden and define the services offered to children with special needs. Table 11.1 provides a historical perspective on the laws that have affected students with special needs.

Table 11.1

Timeline of Major Legislation Affecting Students With Special Needs

1791	Tenth Amendment of the U.S. Constitution gives individual states authority in educational matters.
1880	National Education Association and Office of Education are created and initiate an age-grade-level system categorizing students according to age. Differences in children become apparent quickly.
1919	All states require compulsory school attendance.
1954	U.S. Supreme Court rules on *Brown v. Board of Education of Topeka*, putting an end to "separate but equal" schools. The rights of individual diversity are emphasized and will serve to influence future rulings regarding children with special needs in school.
1961	Special Education Act, P.L. 87–276, authorizes federal money to train teachers of children who are deaf.
1965	Elementary and Secondary Education Act, P.L. 89–10, is the first in a sequence of federal laws to require educational opportunities for students with handicapping conditions.
1973	Section 504 of the Rehabilitation Act, P.L. 93–112, bars discrimination against people with disabilities in any federally funded program and requires appropriate education services for children who are disabled. It mandates access to all public buildings for anyone with a disability.
1975	Education for All Handicapped Children Act, P.L. 94–142, mandates a free and appropriate public education for all children with disabilities. This is the core of funding for special education. It requires that accommodations be made in the public school setting to ensure that educational opportunities are the same for all.
1990	Americans With Disabilities Act, P.L. 101–336, based on the Rehabilitation Act of 1973, is passed and guarantees equal opportunities for persons with disabilities. Physical barriers must be removed, and all new construction must be made accessible to those with disabilities.
1990	Individuals With Disabilities Education Act, P.L. 101–476, formerly the Education for All Handicapped Children Act, expands services and adds additional categories of children eligible to receive services.

Provisions of the ADA and Section 504 Services

Americans With Disabilities Act

The ADA is a broad civil rights law. It protects the rights of all persons with disabilities. Students are eligible if they have a physical or mental impairment that limits one or more major life activities: learning, breathing, walking, eating, and so on. A multidisciplinary accommodation team must be available to determine eligibility. The team then formulates a plan that describes the nature of the disability and how the student is to be accommodated. For instance, accommodations might include hearing devices or medication for allergic reactions or asthma.

Individualized Healthcare Plan

It is up to the school nurse to determine whether a child is in need of an individualized healthcare plan (IHP). Unlike an individualized education plan (IEP), which is mandated by law and educationally based, an IHP is developed solely to provide the nurse a way to recognize healthcare needs, document the provision of care, and progress toward achieving desired outcomes. It simplifies communication with other professionals.

504 Accommodation Plan

Students not meeting the criteria for IDEA services can be considered for services under Section 504 of the Rehabilitation Act of 1973. To be eligible the student must have a physical or mental impairment that substantially limits one or more major life activities—breathing, walking, eating, and so on.

Fast Facts

It is your responsibility to write and update the emergency care plan (ECP) and IHP annually. Books available through your state and national association provide samples you can modify to meet each student's unique needs.

Clinical Snapshot

Jon is a 6-year-old severely diabetic student. His blood sugar levels are unstable, and he needs frequent testing. Emily has developed an IHP that includes an accurate assessment, nursing diagnosis, anticipated outcomes, nursing interventions, and means to evaluate.

(*continued*)

(continued)

Emily then formulates an ECP with specific directions indicating what to do in the event of a school emergency.

If Jon's classification is included in any of the categories under IDEA, the 504 accommodation plan or IHP can be part of the IEP.

Emergency Care Plan

If necessary, an ECP should also be developed to address specific actions to be taken for a child who has a classroom emergency. This plan includes parent and physician contact information and states simply, "If this happens, do this."

Provisions of the IDEA

IDEA provides funding for children with educationally handicapping conditions. Students who fit into one of the following categories of disabilities are eligible for services:

Autism
Deaf–blindness
Deafness
Emotional disturbance
Hearing impairment
Intellectual disability
Multiple disabilities
Orthopedic impairment
Other health impairment
Specific learning disability
Speech/language impairment
Traumatic brain injury
Visual impairment

IDEA reinforces provisions adapted from the Education for All Handicapped Children Act. It includes the following components:

- *A free and appropriate public education for all:* All services must be provided without cost to parents or guardians.
- *The right of due process:* Parents have legal recourse if they are dissatisfied with their children's education.
- *Education in the least restrictive environment:* Mainstreaming, inclusion, and pull-out practices are used to keep the students with special needs in the classroom with peers as much as possible.
- *IEP:* Each child has a specific plan appropriate for his or her needs.

An IEP is written and designed specifically for students with special needs by the child study team. It includes goals and short-term objectives stated in instructional terms. It must include support services to be provided and justification for any special placement recommended. It must be periodically evaluated.

IDEA expanded support services to include transportation; early detection initiatives; related physical, occupational, and speech therapies; and assistive technology devices.

To meet these criteria, districts are required to have a child study team composed of the classroom teacher; the special education teacher; an administrator; a parent or guardian; a learning disability specialist; a psychologist; a social worker; a physical, speech, or occupational therapist; and the school nurse.

Differences Between IDEA and Section 504

The IDEA requires each state to set up a process to address the law. Section 504 is a civil rights law that prohibits discrimination based on handicaps. Federal funds are provided for children classified under IDEA, whereas no federal funds are provided for 504 accommodations. School districts must bear costs for 504 accommodations. All students who are considered to be disabled under IDEA need some type of accommodation to succeed. They must fit into one of the categories to be eligible for services. These same children will need accommodations that will be covered in their IEPs. IDEA addresses only those with specific conditions. Section 504 addresses all children with handicaps in activities of daily living. See Table 11.2 for additional information.

Table 11.2

Areas of Comparison: IDEA and Section 504

Areas of Comparison	IDEA	Section 504
Federal law	Yes	Yes
Due process	Set up by state	Governed by federal law
Funding	Federal funding	No federal funding; school district bears the cost
Accommodation required	All eligible students must fit into a specific category of disability (IEP); those eligible must be accommodated for specific conditions	All students who are unable to perform one or more activities of daily life must be accommodated

IDEA, Individuals With Disabilities Education Act

Table 11.3

Levels of Special Needs Acuity

Level I	Nursing dependent	Requires nursing care 24 hours a day (e.g., ventilator dependent)
Level II	Medically fragile	Has possibility of life-threatening emergency (e.g., severely diabetic, seizure disorder)
Level III	Medically complex	Requires daily treatment or close monitoring (e.g., asthma, attention deficit hyperactivity disorder)
Level IV	Health concerns	Occasional monitoring (e.g., migraines, eating disorders)

Levels of Acuity (Washington State Model)

Children with special needs may require a greater amount of, and more, specialized nursing care in the school setting than do other children. These children are usually classified under IDEA or have a 504 accommodation plan. They are placed in one of four categories, described in Table 11.3.

Some possible reasons for an increase in the number of children identified as having special needs include the following:

- Improved methods of detection
- Better survival rates for infants at risk
- Increased survival of infants from low-weight multiple births with early developmental issues
- The broadening of diagnostic categories encompassing more children

THE SCHOOL NURSE AS A HEALTH RESOURCE

Working with children with special needs and their parents is probably the greatest challenge faced by school nurses. We have been well trained and can easily tend to their physical needs: catheterizations, tube feedings, medications, nebulizer treatments, and so on. It is the emotional care that is absolutely draining.

The parents may be angry. They might mourn their child's lost potential and their own unfulfilled dreams. Parents are not always happy about what school personnel have to say and may choose to vent their wrath on the school, and the school nurse in particular.

Much of special education is funded by the federal government, but some is not. Even one child can financially burden a district and financially ruin a family. Often, parents have to fight for services, and lawsuits can be involved, creating justifiable tension.

Fast Facts

There is no single correct way of providing care for children with special needs. The school nurse must remain an objective, nonjudgmental, and up-to-date resource and must remember that the best decision is always the one that will provide the best benefit to the child. Be mindful that no one, not even you, will be able to fix the source of the problem.

Clinical Snapshot

School nurse Emily is caught between the parents' wishes and district recommendations for placement of a special needs child. Out-of-district placement, busing, and private placement are extremely expensive for any school district. The district is adamant that the child's needs can be met within district. Emily feels strongly that the child's medical issues are so overwhelming they would best be addressed in an out-of-district placement. Emily makes her feelings known, in writing, to the child study team and works to find a comfortable compromise.

ROLE OF SCHOOL NURSES RELATED TO CHILDREN WITH SPECIAL NEEDS

- Know and understand the laws relevant to special education.
- Establish a comfortable, supportive relationship with parents.
- Identify children with special needs as early as possible.
- Help children with special needs blend into the school community.
- Advocate for these children.
- Develop health-related IEP goals.
- Secure signed, written releases for confidential information.
- Develop and implement 504 accommodation plans, IHPs, and ECPs.
- Serve as a liaison among students, teachers, parents, and healthcare providers.
- Identify and utilize community resources.

- Delegate, train, and supervise paraprofessional staff in the delivery of special nursing procedures according to state and school district policies.
- Get out of your centrally located, well-ventilated office, and . . . "shovel the ramp!"

References

American Nurses Association and National Council of State Boards of Nursing. (2005). *Joint Statement on Delegation*. Retrieved from https://www.ncsbn.org/Delegation_joint_statement_NCSBN-ANA.pdf

Lavoie, R. (2005). *It's so much work to be your friend*. New York, NY: Simon & Schuster.

National Center for Education Statistics. (2017). *Indicators of school crime and safety: 2016*. Retrieved from https://nces.ed.gov/pubs2017/2017064.pdf

World Health Organization. (n.d.). *Disabilities*. Retrieved from http://who.int/topics/disabilities/en/

12

Cultural Diversity

If you have ever read historical memoirs of famous generals, you can appreciate how carefully war plans are made. Prior to any battle, extensive research goes into understanding the enemy's religion, ethnicity, and all other aspects of the culture. A plan is formulated, the ground force is established, war is waged, and, hopefully, the opponent is defeated. Only by thinking like the enemy can the war be won. School nurses, as generals leading the struggle for the success of all our children, we have the responsibility to mobilize all school resources to help prepare and protect children from the enemies they will face.

Immigrant families arrive in this country with enemies. These enemies are in the form of risk factors such as poverty, social isolation, language barriers, different lifestyles, and few, if any, extended family members to support them. All of these can impede a child's ability to learn. They can win over the child and prevent him or her from thriving unless our society can help to overcome their virulent influence.

School is where these different students meet and ideally learn with—and about—each other. It is essential that school personnel respect diversity and celebrate the richness that cultural, racial, and ethnic diversity brings to the school.

In this chapter, you will learn:

1. Definitions of *culture* and *diversity*
2. The benefits and challenges of cultural diversity in American schools
3. Cultural sensitivity and competency for diverse school populations
4. Steps to foster academic achievement for students with diverse backgrounds

CULTURE

Culture cannot be defined in just a few words; numerous theories and models have been developed over the years. However, to summarize, culture is:

- Learned behavior that guides thinking, decisions, and activities in a predictable way
- Shared patterns of beliefs, values, and actions
- An inclusive term that covers ethnicity, race, national origin, and religion
- Various traditions that are shared and passed along
- A guide for dealing with other people
- A means to pass values from one generation to another
- A group of students who share the same interests within the class structure; artists, athletes, cheerleaders, and musicians, for example, might be considered separate cultural groups

The first most basic need of all people is to belong. In meeting this need, we also want our culturally different students to keep the essence of who they are and where they came from.

As our country continues to become ever more culturally and ethnically diverse, so do our schools. Therefore, within any large school, there are many different ethnic groups, various languages spoken, and unique cultural attitudes toward education. As the blending of people of different ethnic and racial backgrounds increases in the years to come, it is projected that today's minority populations will become the majority.

At issue today is how to meet the educational needs of so many culturally diverse children. Extremely poor minority children might be at risk for learning disabilities as a result of deprivation or emotional trauma. However, the vast majority of them are perfectly capable of learning as other children do. It is not the ability that they lack; it is the rich experiences that so many other children are afforded in this country today.

Lack of understanding on the part of educators, inadequate communication, and inaccurate evaluations may lead us to label minority students unfairly. School professionals frequently fail to understand and respect different cultural traditions and lack the wisdom to work effectively with various ethnic groups. Schools must remain safe havens for all, regardless of how we differ.

Healthy People 2020 Objectives:
Educational and Community-Based Programs, 14.2:
Increase the inclusion of cultural diversity content in undergraduate nursing programs from 98% in 2009 to 100%.

DIVERSITY

Diversity is a good thing, provided we develop understanding and respect for one another's differences. The goals are to recognize and appreciate the differences, establish helping relationships, and see to it that every child succeeds academically and emotionally finds a comfortable place in the school environment.

Diversity exists in almost every classroom in any school in this country. There are students from different states, countries, and cultures. *Diversity* simply means that differences exist. Differences can include the following:

- Race
- Language
- Ethnicity
- Sexual orientation
- Level or type of education
- Nationality
- Hobbies or interests
- Religion
- Socioeconomic status
- Thinking processes

Fast Facts

As the community is diverse, so will be your schools. And just as the community climate of acceptance influences the school, so, too, does the school influence the community.

(continued)

(*continued*)

Clinical Snapshot

Sanjay is a fourth-grade student who recently immigrated from India. School nurse Susan notices that he refuses to eat lunch in school. He is qualified for a free lunch program but brings a brown bag that is never opened. After questioning Sanjay, Susan finds that he dislikes the cafeteria offerings and is afraid others will laugh at what he brings from home. Susan arranges for him to eat at the same table as another Indian student who is familiar with his food choices and where he can gradually grow more accustomed to the American diet.

Demographics

In the six decades since the U.S. Supreme Court handed down its decision in *Brown v. Board of Education of Topeka* requiring schools to be integrated, a new racial and ethnic landscape has evolved, and the nation's schools have also evolved along with it.

Today's school is less dominated by non-Hispanic Whites than it was in 1950. It is predicted by the U.S. Census Bureau that by the year 2060, we will become a plurality nation, with no one race in the majority (*Education Week*, 2014).

Experts predict that most future immigrants will arrive from Asia and Latin America, and they will continue to settle in metropolitan areas such as New York, Los Angeles, and Chicago. These cities, and many others, include tremendous diversity in cultures, economic status, educational levels, and family values. This is where the challenge begins.

BENEFITS OF CULTURAL DIVERSITY IN SCHOOLS

In a proper school setting, with capable, enthusiastic teachers, there are many benefits to having diverse student populations, as described in the following list:

- *Students are more accepting of differences:* When students learn in a diverse environment at an early age, they become more tolerant and accepting.
- *Students experience freedom from prejudices:* By working together, side by side every day, children learn not to form prejudices or feelings of superiority.
- *Education is promoted and enhanced:* Children learn from each other. They learn cultural tolerance and acceptance as well as academics.

- *Students experience minimum adjustment issues:* When they have been exposed to different cultures at an early age, children are prepared for life beyond school and in an ever more blended world.
- *Patriotism is promoted for all:* When students have the opportunity to learn about other cultures, ideally, they compare and appreciate the learning opportunities that they have been allowed to have in this country (Greater Good Magazine, 2018).

CHALLENGES OF CULTURAL DIVERSITY IN SCHOOLS

Integrating diverse cultures is a challenge. To be successful, some issues must be addressed within a school environment, such as those described in the following list:

- *Teachers' attitudes:* Teachers and other staff members must be willing to extend themselves to address the unique needs of each student.
- *Classroom atmosphere*: Every classroom should be culturally responsive to the needs of all students.
- *Administrative support:* Teachers need support to help communicate with students and parents. Any necessary additional services (interpreters, counselors, etc.) should be provided to them.
- *Proper screening and evaluation procedures:* The multidisciplinary team must be sensitive to every family's needs and flexible in its approach.
- *Staff training*: Education must be provided to all staff members who have contact with culturally diverse students.
- *School and community environment:* Prejudice leading to bullying that escalates to violence is a very real threat to minority students. Members of the school and community must be aware of this and seek to minimize or eliminate this type of threat.
- *Financial burden for school districts:* Without question, the multiple needs of minority students place a financial burden on school districts. Preventive initiatives such as preschool programs and counseling are less costly than intervention programs. These must be offered at any cost by the school district or the state or federal government.

CULTURAL SENSITIVITY AND COMPETENCY

Cultural sensitivity can be defined as having an open attitude toward a culture or ethnic background different from one's own. It is a prerequisite to cultural competence. Cultural competency is the ability to interact effectively with people of other cultures, which grows out of an understanding of and respect for the culture, beliefs, and practices of other people. Because cultural competency is a process, it is enhanced and increased as we grow and learn in our profession.

Steps Toward Cultural Competency

- Self-reflection
- Attaining information about different cultures
- Developing respect and understanding
- Remaining nonjudgmental
- Revising methods of dealing with students as needed

Fast Facts

Some school personnel never achieve cultural competence. Know who these individuals are. Continue to advocate for your students.

Clinical Snapshot

Mrs. G., a third grade teacher who has taught for decades, repeatedly complains about the increasing number of non-English-speaking students. Susan feels sorry for the students placed in her class.

Teachers can become frustrated when trying to communicate with non-English-speaking students and parents. Recommend that non-English-speaking students be placed with teachers who are more understanding. Ensure that interpreters are available when you take a medical history or a parent–teacher conference is planned.

Barriers to Cultural Competency

- *Language:* If necessary, a school district must employ an interpreter to facilitate communication.
- *Ethnic and religious practices:* These may interfere with school policies and expectations.
- *A child's previous experiences:* A child may have witnessed violence or extreme poverty, which will likely affect his or her ability to learn. This must be addressed through counseling.

STEPS TO FOSTER ACADEMIC ACHIEVEMENT

- Keep students in school. Preventing failure is a major step in helping students avoid poverty and issues of low self-worth.
- Encourage attendance at preschool programs. These years are important in building a learning foundation and identifying children with special needs early so that intervention can be started.
- Make sure children are evaluated fairly and without any bias.
- Work as a team with other professionals in the community and school district.
- Help students to connect with the school, staff, and other students.
- Encourage staff education.

Role of School Nurses in Dealing With Culturally Diverse Students

- Reflect on your own feelings regarding the various cultures of students.
- Research information on the various ethnic groups within your school.
- Work toward personally becoming culturally competent.
- Help organize staff educational programs.
- Serve on multidisciplinary teams, and advocate for children from other cultures.
- Serve as a liaison among school, students, and parents.
- Help promote an atmosphere of respect, cooperation, and acceptance throughout the school.
- Provide opportunities for students and staff to celebrate cultural pride.
- Continue to offer your office and self as a refuge for all who need a safe place to visit.
- Remain cognizant of the underlying issues of great concern for immigrant children: housing, transportation, access to healthcare, counseling services, poverty, ethnic prejudice, and so on.

References

Education Week. (2014). Data: Race and Ethnicity in U.S. Schools Today. *Education Week, 33*(1), 31. Retrieved from https://www.edweek.org/ew/section/multimedia/data-package-us-schools-racial-ethnic-landscape.html

Greater Good Magazine. (2018). *How students benefit from school diversity. A complex new study strengthens the case for racially balanced schools—and uncovers additional advantages for students of all ethnicities.* Retrieved from https://greatergood.berkeley.edu/article/item/how_students_benefit_from_school_diversity

13

Childhood Obesity

The fastest growing epidemic in our country is obesity, affecting all ages with devastating short- and long-term complications. Childhood obesity causes serious risk factors for many major illnesses and unprecedented financial and social costs to our nation. Some health professionals feel that the schools have contributed to the problem with fat- and sugar-laden school lunches, celebrations, vending machine offerings, bake sales, and lack of recess or physical education during the school day. Legislation to combat the rise of obesity has been proposed and implemented to support school districts in offering healthier food choices and more opportunities for physical activity. Today's statistics on obesity are truly alarming. This epidemic requires immediate attention if we are to stem this public health crisis.

The school nurse has the important role of assessing and managing overweight and obese children in the school setting, as well as implementing prevention programs. Part of our task is to look closely at obese students and staff members and recognize the depth of their suffering.

In this chapter, you will learn:

1. The scope of the childhood obesity crisis
2. How to identify children who are obese and overweight
3. Causes of obesity and the emotional components of food
4. Consequences of obesity
5. Preventive programs and support that can be initiated within the school

SCOPE OF THE CHILDHOOD OBESITY CRISIS

According to the Centers for Disease Control and Prevention (CDC, 2018), the prevalence of overweight children in the United States has reached alarming levels. Approximately 13.7 million children and adolescents are considered obese. Statistics clearly show that childhood obesity has more than tripled in the past 30 years. The rate of obesity for children aged 6 to 11 years increased from 6.5% in 1980 to 20.6% in 2018. Adolescents aged 12 to 19 years showed a similar increase, from 5% to 18%. Hispanics (25.8%) and non-Hispanic Blacks (22.0%) had higher obesity prevalence than non-Hispanic Whites. Sadly, it appears that childhood obesity is a trend that will continue growing unless steps are immediately taken to get it under control.

Healthy People 2020 Objective 10.3: Nutrition and Weight Status:
Reduce the proportion of children and adolescents aged 12 to 19 years who are considered obese from 17.9% to 16.1%.

Physical Activity, 4.1–4.3
Increase the proportion of the nation's public and private schools that require daily physical education for all students:
Elementary—from 3.8% in 2006 to 4.2%
Middle—from 7.8% in 2006 to 8.6%
High—from 2.1% in 2006 to 2.3%

Physical Activity, 6.2
Increase the proportion of school districts that require regularly scheduled elementary school recess from 57.1% in 2006 to 62.8%.

IDENTIFYING OVERWEIGHT OR OBESE CHILDREN

Simply put, when a person is overweight or obese, there is an excess of body fat. The person is taking in more calories than his or her level of activity requires. Excess calories are stored as fat in the body. If overconsumption of calories is persistent, fat accumulates, causing weight gain.

Fast Facts

Obese children may be rejected by their peers and will cope by simply eating more. Society's attitude toward these individuals is

(*continued*)

(continued)

probably the one type of prejudice still tolerated within schools, communities, and the nation itself.

Clinical Snapshot

Consuela is a 12-year-old sixth-grade student, who was adopted at birth from Central America. She is 62 inches tall, weighs 230 pounds, is hypertensive (blood pressure [BP] of 160/100), and has a body mass index (BMI) over 95%. Untidy and socially isolated, she is a very unhappy young girl. Previous attempts by the school nurse, Mary Ellen, to communicate concern to the parents proved unsuccessful and produced angry accusations of intrusiveness. As graduation to middle school approached, Consuela became even heavier and developed school phobia, refusing most days to get out of bed. Mom has now asked for help.

A problem must be acknowledged before change can take place. The school nurse is now in a position to help this family. Consuela should be referred for a comprehensive physical examination, and an individualized healthcare plan should be developed.

The first step in determining whether a child is overweight or obese is to calculate his or her BMI. This is the quickest and easiest screening tool. School nurses check students' height and weight annually. From these numbers, the BMI of each student can be calculated. BMI is determined by using the following formula (CDC, 2014):

$$\text{weight (lb)}/[\text{height (in.)}]^2 \times 703$$

The number obtained is then referenced on the CDC's BMI-for-age growth charts for girls and boys (www.cdc.gov/growthcharts). The acceptable amount of body fat changes with age and differs for boys and girls. Where a child's BMI falls on the graph determines the level of concern for the child:

- Underweight: Less than the 5th percentile
- Healthy weight: 5th percentile to less than the 85th percentile
- Overweight: 85th percentile to less than the 95th percentile
- Obese: Equal to or greater than the 95th percentile
- For the purposes of this chapter, the terms *obesity* and *overweight* are used interchangeably

CAUSES OF CHILDHOOD OBESITY

As noted by Bellows and Moore (2013), many variables can cause obesity, including those listed in the following sections. Frequently, these variables interact to create even greater problems for obese children.

Genetics

Certain people are simply more susceptible to weight gain. We can see clearly that obesity runs in families. Parental obesity is a strong predictor for child obesity.

Behavior

Some behaviors contribute to weight gain. These include eating an unhealthful diet, limited engagement in physical activities, and having a sedentary lifestyle.

Diet

- Reliance on fast foods
- Preference for high-sugar snacks and drinks
- Use of large portion sizes
- Use of food as a reward
- Few meals eaten with family

Activities

- Excessive screen time (e.g., watching television, working at computer, playing video games)
- Little or no participation in sports
- Fewer children walking to and from school

Lifestyle

- Sedentary lifestyle
- Frequent snacking on junk foods

Environment

The home and school setting may both contribute to obesity. Children with working parents may be told to wait for their parents at the public library or to go directly home, lock the door, and stay inside until a parent arrives home. They may not be permitted to play outside unsupervised for safety reasons. This contributes to boredom, snacking, and lack of physical activity.

Sociodemographics

Families with low-income levels may not be able to provide their children with healthful choices such as fresh fruits and vegetables. Bagged snacks like potato chips and cookies do not spoil and are cheaper.

EMOTIONAL COMPONENTS OF FOOD

Rimm (2004) explained that food means different things to different people. To understand the meanings that food may have for an obese child, consider the following emotional components.

Food Is Love

- Babies are conditioned to equate food with love. If an infant cries or is cranky, we feed him or her. We offer milk, cookies, juice, cereal, or whatever it takes to make the baby stop crying.
- Therefore, if food is love, does the withdrawal of food mean the baby is not loved?

Food Is Health

- We consider a chubby baby to be healthy. Small children are encouraged to eat so they grow "strong and healthy."
- If we feed them less, does that mean they are not healthy?

Food Is Celebration

- Every time people of all cultures gather in joy, we celebrate with food. This means that birthdays, holidays, a new job, graduation, wedding, and so on all justify eating. The more important the occasion, the more elaborate the food.
- If we eat less rich food, does the occasion have less significance?

Food Is Basic

- We simply love to eat! It satisfies our basic need for nourishment and gives us great pleasure. Most Americans can afford to eat as much and as often as they wish, and that is exactly what we do.
- So, because we can afford food, why cannot we eat what we want?

Food Is Social Status

- Many important interviews and celebrations are held at expensive restaurants. Guests are entertained lavishly at dinners in four- and five-star restaurants with elite clientele who can afford the best.
- Do we not deserve this too?

Food Is Power

- Some children control the dinner table by refusing to eat or by gorging themselves. They use food to manipulate their parents into bribing them: "Just finish what is on your plate, and then you can have a present."
- Is it not important to get the child to eat using any means possible?

Food Can Become a Problem

- Parents rejoice when the pediatrician announces that their child is thriving and has attained high growth and weight percentages. At some point, however, this can become a problem for parents who realize that their child is becoming obese.
- Why cannot we be complacent in this situation?

CONSEQUENCES OF OBESITY

The physical and psychosocial consequences of childhood obesity are frightening, both in the short term and the long term (see Table 13.1).

Table 13.1

Physical and Psychosocial Consequences of Childhood Obesity and Duration of Impact

Physical Consequences	Duration of Impact
Adult obesity	Long term
Gallbladder disease	Long term
Heart disease and hypertension	Long and short term
Hyperlipidemia	Long term
Diabetes mellitus type 2	Long term
Early sexual maturation	Short term
Asthma	Long and short term
Sleep disturbances (e.g., apnea)	Long and short term

(continued)

Table 13.1

Physical and Psychosocial Consequences of Childhood Obesity and Duration of Impact (*continued*)

Physical Consequences	Duration of Impact
Musculoskeletal diseases	Long term
Depression	Long and short term
Social ineptness	Long and short term
Victim of bullying	Long and short term
Poor body image	Long and short term
Reduced quality of life	Long and short term
Low academic achievement	Long and short term
Poor school attendance	Short term

Fast Facts

Each state develops its own curriculum content standards. These address the subject to be taught, and at what grade level, as well as strategies to help students develop skills to reduce high-risk health-related behaviors. The curriculum standards are vaguely written, allowing teachers to individualize lessons to meet the needs of the student and class. If obesity is prevalent in a particular class, lessons should be focused accordingly.

Clinical Snapshot

When school nurse Mary Ellen reviewed the entire class's BMI statistics, she noted that Consuela was not the only obese child in her class. Therefore, a broader approach needed to be taken. Mary Ellen sat down with the classroom teacher and altered the health curriculum to focus more on proper food intake and the importance of exercise.

SCHOOL INITIATIVES TO PREVENT CHILDHOOD OBESITY

Childhood obesity is best addressed by using each of the eight components of the Coordinated School Health Program.

Coordinated School Health Program

1. *Health education:* In this organized, sequential K–12 plan for delivering information, students are given relevant information

about diet and diseases throughout their school experience. This helps them make wise health decisions based on factual information. Education is the first step in prevention, and it is most effective.

2. *Physical education:* This component is a planned, sequential K–12 curriculum that provides cognitive content and experiences in a variety of activities, including basic movement skills, physical fitness, rhythm and dance, and individual and team sports. This component is especially important for students who are not physically active outside of school.
3. *School health services:* These services include the school nurse's role in measuring each student's height and weight to determine his or her BMI. This is how overweight children are identified, and steps to help them are initiated.
4. *Nutrition services:* These include services that provide students with nutritionally balanced, varied meals and healthful snacks in an atmosphere that promotes social interaction. All students should have only nutritious choices available during the school hours. This includes breakfast/lunch offerings, classroom celebrations, and vending machine options.
5. *Counseling, psychological, and social services:* These are services that offer broad-based individual and group assessments, interventions, and referrals that attend to the mental, emotional, and social needs of students. Obese students may need more services than can be offered at school. Referrals to appropriate outside agencies may be warranted.
6. *Healthful and safe school environment:* A healthful and safe school environment is one that is free of prejudice against people who are obese and supports every person's need for acceptance and belonging within the school community. Recess time should be enjoyed by all with participation in noncompetitive physical activities.
7. *Health promotion for staff:* Health promotion programs such as health screenings, assessments, health education, and physical activities are important for the wellness and morale of staff. Teachers must be well themselves before they can effectively teach students.
8. *Parent/family and community involvement:* Schools need to partner with parents and community groups to address the needs of obese students. Obesity is often a problem for siblings and parents as well, and informed, involved parents can greatly help obese children. Often, community agencies sponsor health-related activities in which these children can participate.

Fast Facts

When talking with the family of an obese child, the topic of weight must be handled sensitively. Parents may be offended and feel you are intruding. Obesity may very well be only a symptom of a greater problem. Tread lightly in this area as parents may be defensive. Recognize and seek professional help for morbidly obese children or adults.

Clinical Snapshot

Consuela's mom immediately became defensive when she received the referral letter that her daughter brought home the day after school nurse Mary Ellen conducted height and weight screenings at school. A better approach might have been for Mary Ellen to make a phone call letting the mother know that she would be getting the BMI referral in the mail shortly. An explanation of school policy and your sincere concern may soften a parent's irate reaction.

ROLE OF SCHOOL NURSES IN SUPPORTING THOSE WHO ARE OVERWEIGHT

- Check each student's, height, weight, and BMI annually, and make referrals as necessary.
- Organize a group of concerned students, staff, and parents to work with you on preventive programs such as health clubs, walking groups, weight monitoring, teacher–student buddy system, and so on.
- Educate students, parents, and staff about the immediate and long-term effects of childhood obesity.
- Create opportunities for the use of school gyms, weight rooms, and playground areas outside of school hours.
- Support local, state, and federal obesity prevention programs.
- Address the issues of healthful diets and exercise through the comprehensive school health curriculum.
- Assess the school's current health policy and procedures. Seek to update and improve them as necessary.
- Evaluate and implement changes in school lunch and party policies.
- Evaluate and implement changes in food catering menus and vending machine offerings.

- Be part of community efforts outside of school to enhance healthful lifestyles.
- Develop 504 or individualized healthcare plans as needed for obese students.
- Encourage such events as "Health Food Sales" or "Salad Days" as fundraisers instead of candy sales.
- Encourage outdoor play at recess, gym, and lunchtimes.
- Celebrate the individual's strengths. Look at the total child.
- In providing health counseling, attempt to coach, rather than judge.
- Focus on lifestyle changes rather than diet alone.
- Be a role model.

References

Bellows, L., & Moore, R. (2013, March). *Childhood obesity.* Retrieved from https://extension.colostate.edu/docs/pubs/foodnut/09317.pdf

Centers for Disease Control and Prevention. (2014). *About BMI for children and teens.* Retrieved from www.cdc.gov/healthyweight/assessing/bmi/childrens_bmi/about_childrens_bmi.html

Centers for Disease Control and Prevention. (2018). *Obesity and overweight.* Retrieved from https://www.cdc.gov/nchs/fastats/obesity-overweight.htm

Rimm, S. (2004). *Rescuing the emotional lives of overweight children* (pp. 6–25, 45–51). New York, NY: St. Martin's Press.

14

Autism Spectrum Disorders

It is increasingly clear that schools today are becoming the primary site for detection, intervention, and treatment of a variety of illnesses. This is especially true for mental health issues. No matter how loving or intelligent a child's parents are, this is a painful area. Parents often delay seeking help and find it difficult, if not impossible, to be objective about their own child.

It would be most helpful if there were a clear definition, known cause, and specific treatments for autism. Unfortunately, this information does not yet exist. The body of knowledge is growing, but for now, we must examine what we do know and continue to identify children with autism as early as possible so that they have the best possible prognosis.

In this chapter, you will learn:

1. The definition of *autism*, along with a history of the disorder, causal theories, and risk factors
2. Classifications of autism and statistics relating to incidence
3. Signs and symptoms of children with autism
4. Possible comorbid disorders and differential diagnoses
5. School interventions and how to maintain an active role in supporting children with autism, their siblings, and parents

Healthy People 2020 Objective:
Maternal, Infant, and Child Health, 29.1:
Increase the proportion of children (aged 10–35 months) who have been screened for an autism spectrum disorder (ASD) and other developmental delays from 22.6% in 2007 to 24.9%.

DEFINITION OF AUTISM

Autism is an umbrella term used to describe a group of intricate developmental brain disorders known as *pervasive developmental disorders*. Autism is a spectrum disorder, which means that all autistic children share some common symptoms but these vary in severity, specificity, and behavior, with overlapping and considerable individual variation. For our purposes, *autism spectrum disorder* and *pervasive developmental disorders* are terms that can be used interchangeably.

Autism spectrum disorder cuts across all lines of socioeconomic status, educational background, race, religion, and ethnicity. It is definitely not caused by a lack of maternal nurturing, as previously thought. Most experts would also state that it is not caused by immunizations, though some still cling to this belief.

The Individuals With Disabilities Education Act (IDEA) has identified autism as one of the areas included for services and mandates that every autistic child receive a free, appropriate education in the least restrictive environment. This places an enormous financial burden on the local school districts. It also places an enormous emotional burden on the school nurse.

HISTORY OF AUTISM

In 1938, child psychiatrist Leo Kanner, working out of Johns Hopkins Hospital in Baltimore, Maryland, evaluated 11 children with similarities that he had never seen before. He published his findings in an article entitled "Autistic Disturbances of Affective Contact." Kanner described these children as viewing people as unwelcome intruders in their world, and as being detached and inaccessible. He believed that they lived in a world of their own, where they could not be reached. Kanner used the word *autistic* because he was struck by the children's self-absorption (Bruey, 2004, pp. 30–31).

Fast Facts

The word *autism* was also used for people diagnosed with schizophrenia, and many once believed that these were related conditions. Today it is known that the two diseases are separate. Autistic behaviors are easily recognized by the trained observer.

Clinical Snapshot

Mr. and Mrs. Smith have two children. The older daughter is a third-grade student in your school. You have noticed that the preschool-aged younger brother does not maintain eye contact, will not socialize, and engages in repetitive play. He does not attend any preschool program, and you are concerned. School nurse Donna suggests to the parents that he be evaluated by the child study team.

CAUSAL THEORIES AND RISK FACTORS

The etiology of autism is still unknown, but it is theorized that, because the disorder involves such a wide spectrum of symptoms, there are most likely many causes. It is believed that an autistic child's brain handles information differently from the way other children's brains do.

Recent evidence suggest that autism may be caused by:

- Random genetic mutations, as it is associated with advanced parental age at conception
- Failure of the embryonic cells to undergo normal patterns of migration during early development, causing defects in brain structure and wiring of nerve-cell circuits that control social, language, and other abilities
- Fetal exposure to abnormally high levels of testosterone in utero since autism affects mostly males (Psychology Today, 2019)

There are probably a variety of other factors that increase the likelihood of a child being in the spectrum of autism, including environmental, biological, and genetic factors. It is generally agreed that autism is a developmental disability and that its basis is organic with a genetic component.

Fast Facts

Very few diagnoses are feared as much as autism. Helping families of autistic children recognize, accept, and cope with the diagnosis will be the most difficult challenge you meet.

Clinical Snapshot

Once Donna, the school nurse, makes the recommendation for a referral, she must continue to support the parent through the process. Donna may have to deal with resentment on the part of the parent. If a child is found to have behaviors that place him or her within the spectrum, much work will need to be done as early as possible. Early detection and intervention are imperative.

FACTORS INFLUENCING AUTISM

- Genetic predisposition
- A sibling with autism
- Male preponderance
- Presence of another genetic disorder
- Maternal use of certain drugs during pregnancy

AREAS OF CONCERN

Autistic children have deficits in three core areas: social skills, communication, and behavior or interests. Because there is no specific blood test or other diagnostic tool, the diagnosis must be based on behavior, which varies considerably, especially with very young children (Table 14.1). In addition, these children may experience fine or gross motor delays or cognitive issues.

CLASSIFICATIONS OF AUTISM SPECTRUM DISORDERS

There are five recognized types of autism spectrum disorders (Table 14.2).

STATISTICS

On April 26, 2018, the Centers for Disease Control and Prevention (CDC) released new data on the prevalence of autism in the United

Table 14.1

Deficits and Associated Behaviors of Autistic Children

Deficit	Behavior
Social skills	Impairment in nonverbal behavior (eye-to-eye contact, facial expressions, gestures) Failure to develop appropriate peer relationships; lack of spontaneously sharing enjoyment and ideas Lack of emotional reciprocity (acting as if in own world)
Communication	Delay in, or lack of development of, spoken language with no attempt to compensate Marked impairment initiating or sustaining a conversation with others who can speak Echolalia or pronominal reversal (instead of "I want a drink," it is "Peter wants a drink") Lack of varied spontaneous make-believe play or social imitative play that is age appropriate
Behavior or interests	Preoccupation with parts or objects Behaviors that are narrow in their focus and repetitive Inflexible adherence to routines and rituals Stereotyped and repetitive motor mannerisms (hand or finger flapping, complex body movements)

Table 14.2

Recognized Types of Autism Spectrum Disorders and Their Manifestations

Type	Manifestations
1. Autistic disorder (classic)	Significant language delay Social and communication impairment Unusual behaviors and interests Intellectual disability Most common type
2. Asperger's syndrome	Higher functioning form of autism Less pronounced social challenges Idiosyncratic social skills and play Typical language development Average or above-average intellect
3. Childhood disintegrative disorder	Typical development for first 2 years Regression then occurs between 2 and 4 years Developmental behaviors affected: socializing, motor skills, toilet training, use of nonverbal behaviors Very rare disorder

(*continued*)

Table 14.2

Recognized Types of Autism Spectrum Disorders and Their Manifestations (*continued*)

Type	Manifestations
4. Rett syndrome	Affects only girls Mildly delayed as infants By 18 months, have progressive loss of skill in gross motor skills, language, and social areas Growth of head circumference slows Difficult gait and balance Repetitive hand-wringing and hyperventilating behaviors are common
5. Pervasive developmental disorder: not otherwise specified	This category is considered when there is severe impairment in social skills and verbal communication, but the criteria are not met for another specific area

States. This surveillance study identified one in 59 children (one in 37 boys and one in 151 girls) as having autism spectrum disorder.

This rate appears to be increasing by 10% to 17% annually. The reason for this dramatic increase is not clear, but most would agree that there are now better means of detection and the definition of *autism* has been broadened to include many additional conditions. Regardless of the cause, there are more children with autism than with cancer, diabetes, and AIDS combined (Autism Speaks, 2018).

SIGNS AND SYMPTOMS

Most parents recall starting to be concerned when the child is about 1 year of age. Severe problems can be noted earlier, whereas some children may not demonstrate deficits until closer to 2 years. Children's development may appear to be age appropriate until 18 to 24 months and then cease to progress.

Usually, autism is diagnosed around age 3 and will be a lifelong condition. Early signs to watch for include the following:

- Not responding to name by 12 months
- Not pointing to objects of interest by 14 months
- Not playing pretend games by 18 months
- Avoiding eye contact

- Difficulty understanding feelings, their own or others
- Delayed speech and language skills
- Echolalia
- Spinning, rocking, and flapping
- Sensory issues (CDC, 2006)

THE FAMILY

As with all other major health issues, the family of an autistic child is significantly affected. Parents often go through stages of denial, fear, anger, and panic, and their concerns are indeed warranted. At best, they must be prepared for a lifetime of challenges with the very real possibility that their child may never be fully independent. The school nurse will play an important role as parents go through the process of acceptance of their child's special needs. The school nurse can be of even greater help with any siblings.

Be mindful of the impact this diagnosis has on the entire family. Parents tend to focus on the child with the greatest needs and can unintentionally neglect the other children. The family may experience financial difficulties if one parent needs to stay at home to be available for physician visits and various therapies. Stress may cause marital unrest and even further pain for the other children. Seek out these siblings, and support their needs as well.

COMORBID DISORDERS

A number of disorders are associated with autism spectrum disorder. These disorders can overlap. Alone, they cannot be diagnostic of autism; however, the school nurse needs to be mindful of the possibility of their presence.

Some Comorbid Disorders Associated With Autism

- Seizures
- Immune system dysfunction
- Hyperactivity
- Anxiety
- Gastrointestinal disorders
- Allergies
- Obsessive behaviors
- Depression

DIFFERENTIAL DIAGNOSES

Often, children with autism have more than one problem. Multiple issues can become apparent and take various forms and different combinations. One issue can easily exacerbate another, so each must be addressed and handled appropriately.

The school nurse needs to be aware that when a diagnosis of autism spectrum disorder has been made, the following conditions must be considered as well to determine their possible influence on the child's behavior:

- Speech and language disorders; aphasia
- Social phobia
- Central auditory processing disorder
- Mentally challenged
- Oppositional defiant disorder
- Hearing impairment
- Chromosomal or metabolic disorders
- Attention deficit disorder
- Learning disability
- Sensory integration dysfunction
- Anxiety; obsessive-compulsive disorder
- Tourette syndrome
- Depression
- Bipolar disorder

SCHOOL INTERVENTIONS

Schools can take a number of steps to help children with autism.

- Early detection
  - *Preschool programs have afforded professionals the opportunity to see children at younger ages. This allows us to detect problems and intervene early. The sooner a child is diagnosed and treated, the better the outcome will be.*
  - *Siblings of diagnosed children must be assessed as early as possible because they may also have a genetic component predisposing them to autism.*
- Child study team involvement
  - *A team approach is needed for speech, occupational, and physical therapy. Children who need such therapy, if necessary, are placed in a self-contained classroom.*
  - *Behavior modification, communication therapy, and social skills development are essential.*

- Intervention strategies
    - *The classroom environment must be structured.*
    - *The teacher must be educated about the specific needs of the autistic child.*
    - *The teacher should develop consistent, predictable routines and schedules.*
    - *The teacher should determine the child's learning style and present new information appropriately.*
    - *Sensory stimulation, such as loud noises, should be limited.*
    - *Peer mentoring and small-group activities with mainstream students should be encouraged.*
    - *Positive reinforcement should be used as much as possible.*

Fast Facts

Before attempting to help families of children with autism, find out what they know and have already been told. Clarify misconceptions, and build on the strengths of the child.

Clinical Snapshot

Mr. and Mrs. Smith have accepted that their son is within the autism spectrum. Mrs. Smith frequently calls to speak with Donna, the school nurse, and asks advice. Donna needs to be careful with what she shares. She needs to check to see what the parents have previously been told by the physician and other members of the child study team and to support her colleagues. If she vehemently disagrees with what a parent has been told, she needs to go back to the source for clarification and have them discuss it with the parent.

ROLE OF THE SCHOOL NURSE IN HELPING CHILDREN WITH AUTISM AND THEIR FAMILIES

- Encourage the development of and attendance in preschool programs in your district to facilitate early detection.
- Be alert for signs and symptoms of autism spectrum disorder in children, especially if one sibling has already been diagnosed.

- Actively participate in Intervention and Referral Services or child study team meetings, or both, to identify and plan the program for these children.
- In working with the parents, attempt to determine their level of knowledge, perspective, and coping skills regarding their child's diagnosis. Build on this information.
- Prepare the medical component for the individualized education plan.
- Prepare the individualized healthcare plan, 504 accommodation plan, or emergency care plan, as needed.
- Be mindful that comorbid diseases and differential diagnoses are possible.
- Serve as a health resource and liaison for staff, family, and student.
- Consider referral to outside community agencies when warranted.
- Be especially attentive to siblings. Their needs may go unrecognized while parents attempt to cope.

References

Autism Speaks. (2018). *What is autism?* Retrieved from https://www.autismspeaks.org/what-autism

Bruey, C. T. (2004). *Demystifying autism spectrum disorders: A guide to diagnosis for parents and professionals* (pp. 45–80). Bethesda, MD: Woodbine House.

Centers for Disease Control and Prevention. (2006). *Facts about ASD.* Retrieved from http://www.cdc.gov/ncbddd/autism/facts.html

Psychology Today. (2019). *Autism spectrum disorder.* Retrieved from https://www.psychologytoday.com/us/conditions/autism-spectrum-disorder

15

Adolescent Sexuality

Adolescence marks the passage from child to adult. It is considered the most crucial stage in human lives. One's physical appearance changes dramatically, and the brain evolves further. Adolescents have the opportunity to begin to prioritize responsibilities so they can make good decisions and become fully functioning, productive adults.

Each child goes through many rapid changes in growth—physically, socially, emotionally, and intellectually—as he or she begins to develop more advanced thinking skills in preparation for adulthood. The fact that all these changes take place in a relatively short period of time causes confusion and turbulence for adolescents and all who surround them.

Sexual development and curiosity reaches its peak during these years. Many students feel they are different and just do not know why. It is essential that the school nurse be a reliable resource for students, staff, and parents.

In this chapter, you will learn:

1. How the brain develops
2. The stages of adolescence
3. The physical and mental changes common to all adolescents
4. Factors that influence adolescents
5. Sexual health terminology and issues of today's adolescents
6. Strategies the school nurse can use to help identify and treat adolescents experiencing difficulty finding their place in society

THE RAPIDLY CHANGING BODY AND BRAIN

Physiologically, adolescence presents many unique challenges as compared with other growth periods. Physical and mental disturbances increase in proportion to these changes. As a child begins to mature, he or she shows sexual interest, seeks autonomy, is susceptible to growing peer influence, and is expected to achieve academic success. These multiple interchanging influences can cause overwhelming stress, which will have an impact on the educational process. An unhappy, insecure child cannot learn. Basic needs for belonging and acceptance must be met first.

Fast Facts

Today we recognize that there are significant changes as the brain develops. These changes account for the adolescent's unpredictable behavior.

Clinical Snapshot

Josh is sent to sit with the nurse to *cool off.* He refused to cooperate in math class and was rude to his teacher. You sit next to this now sweet 14-year-old and ask what the problem was. Josh tries to explain his poor behavior but seems generally confused himself. School nurse Lisa is constantly amazed by the inconsistencies apparent in teens.

These inconsistencies are seen both between teens and day to day within individual teens. It is not uncommon for a teen to behave appropriately in one setting and quite irrationally in another.

Today's effective diagnostic tools and research allow us to begin to understand the rapid changes in function as the brain continues to mature during adolescence. Brain development progresses from the posterior to the frontal lobes. This latter area, known as the prefrontal cortex, is the portion designated for planning and recognizing consequences. It is the last part of the brain to develop.

The prefrontal cortex communicates with the rest of the brain through connections called *synapses*. A tremendous growth in synapses occurs during adolescence. Because children mature at different rates, it is easy to understand why some have more difficulty during this phase of development. Their brains have not yet advanced in the area needed for decision-making (Edmonds, 2010).

Adolescence is also a time when there is an opportunity to establish the skills and values needed for adult life. Most children do just that and find their way with minimal issues. Unfortunately, we most often hear about the negative aspects and behaviors of adolescents. For some, the path to full, productive, adult potential may have obstacles such as illness, frequent moves, the death of a loved one, or a family financial crisis. Everyday problems can turn into large ones or into complex disorders that cloud the path and add to the stress that a child is experiencing.

The school nurse's role is to recognize the struggling students and to clear and illuminate the path as we guide them along. If the path is totally blocked, a student will need an entirely different approach. Sometimes, the alternate path will also have obstacles. A student can be misdiagnosed, experience ineffective treatment, have additional issues that were overlooked, or have parents who are reluctant to seek help altogether. Even the best-educated, loving parent can fail to recognize or accept the seriousness of an adolescent's problems.

The goal, of course, is to recognize a lost child early and provide him or her with a safe, accepting path to adulthood. It is essential to identify an obstacle before it becomes an overwhelming disorder. Once the school nurse helps such a child find the correct path, it can lead to full, productive, adult behavior, and the student can reach his or her full potential.

Fast Facts

Adolescence commences around age 10 years and ends between 18 and 24 years. Some experts divide adolescence into stages: early—10 to 13 years; middle—14 to 17; and late—18 to 24 years.

Clinical Snapshot

Twelve-year-old Keisha and her younger brother are in the sole custody of her dad. The mother is incarcerated with little chance of obtaining freedom. Aware of this, school nurse Lisa speaks with Keisha's dad and, with his permission, offers to talk privately with her about menstruation and other anticipated bodily changes.

As students progress from one stage to another, there can be confusion. In school, they are surrounded by peers dealing with their own unrest, while at home, they may be alone in going through this tumultuous time. When there is little or no support at home, the school nurse can be available to help.

STAGES OF ADOLESCENCE

Adolescence is divided into three stages: early, middle, and late (Table 15.1).

Table 15.1

Stages of Adolescence and Associated Typical Behaviors

Stage	Age	Typical Behaviors
Early	10–13	Thinks in concrete terms; can categorize thoughts into usable forms; little consideration of long-term consequences Behavior may be rebellious, defiant of adult authority Lacks self-esteem Attempts to seek own identity; begins to question family values Influenced significantly by peers, uses peer-group "language," adopts peer-group clothing style
Middle	14–17	Thinking is more abstract; begins to think of, and be concerned about, long-term consequences Increasing interest in sex Continues to develop definition of self, especially with intimate relationships; concerns over physical and sexual attractiveness May experiment with drugs (cigarettes, alcohol, marijuana) and sex Moodiness Seeks greater independence from family, may complain that family interferes, seeks privacy from family Tests rules and behavioral limits
Late	18–20	Begins to make independent choices Seeks additional responsibilities Establishes relationship with a significant other Finds employment or goes to college

Sources: Adapted from Selekman, J. (Ed.). (2013). *School nursing: A comprehensive text* (pp. 2–14, 64, 1216–1243, 257–281, 407–435, 943–959, 970–997, 1135–1136). Philadelphia: F.A. Davis (p. 369–378); Scudder, L. E. (2006). Pediatric growth and development. In S. M. Nettina (Ed.), *Lippincott's manual of nursing practice* (8th ed.). Philadelphia: Lippincott Williams & Wilkins (p. 1319); Garber, B. D. (2010). *Developmental psychology for family law professionals.* New York: Springer Publishing Company (p. 58, 73); and American Academy of Child and Adolescent Psychiatry. (2004). *Facts for families: Normal adolescent development.* Retrieved from www.actforyouth.net/resources/rf/rf_stages_0504.cfm.

ADOLESCENT CHANGES

Physical Maturity

Puberty begins during early adolescence and progresses systematically for both boys and girls. Each child goes through the various stages according to his or her own pattern. Thus, children of the same grade and age can appear quite different in terms of physical maturation. This can cause some to have a poor body image and lower self-esteem.

Anticipated Appearance and Behaviors

- Significant physical growth
- Appearance of secondary sex characteristics

Behaviors That Are Cause for Concern

- Physical confrontations
- Bullying

Sexual Interest

Adolescence is the time when children begin to show interest in sexual issues and partners. Early experiences consist mostly of thoughts that are not acted upon. During the middle and late adolescent stages, young people seek their sexual identity and begin to form meaningful relationships.

Anticipated Appearance and Behaviors

- Greater interest in sexual issues
- Girls—breast and hip changes; boys—growth in penis and testicles, occurrence of wet dreams

Behaviors That Are Cause for Concern

- Promiscuity
- Unprotected sex

Autonomy

Adolescents urgently seek to be their own person. A close, strong family bond helps to ground them for future changes and decision-making, but separation is clearly a healthy behavior.

Anticipated Appearance or Behaviors

- Questioning adult decisions
- Recognition that parents and teachers are fallible

Behaviors That Are Cause for Concern

- Repeated rule and limit testing
- Withdrawal from family
- School truancy and phobias

Peer Relations

Peer relations are important at this time. Most adolescents care more about what friends think than about what parents think. This is normal and to be expected. During late adolescence, young people begin to seek that one special partner.

Anticipated Appearance or Behaviors

- Desire to be popular with peers
- Self-involvement

Behaviors That Are Cause for Concern

- Partnerships with gangs
- Weapon possession
- Illegal drug use
- Talk of suicide
- Self-injury
- Depression

FACTORS INFLUENCING ADOLESCENCE

There are four factors that significantly influence the adolescent in his or her journey toward adulthood.

1. *Biological influences:* Hormones have a significant impact on physical, emotional, and psychological changes as a child goes through puberty. The appearance of secondary sex characteristics, such as female breast development and male facial hair, can threaten self-image. Some adolescents enjoy their new, grown-up appearances, whereas others become self-conscious and awkward.

Fast Facts

Adolescent issues are areas on which experts are just beginning to focus. It is felt that unrecognized problems at this age can lead to serious adult problems in later years.

(*continued*)

(continued)

Clinical Snapshot

David's family moved numerous times during his high-school years. As soon as he formed friendships, his dad received another transfer. School nurse Lisa notes that David has difficulty establishing peer relationships, is emotionally distant, and appears unhappy. She points this out to his teachers and asks them to join you in monitoring David's socialization. This is discussed at the parent–teacher conference so David's parents are aware of the possible long-term effects on their child.

2. *Cognitive influences:* Adolescents begin to think more rationally. They begin to think in hypothetical terms that extend beyond the here and now. They work hard to develop their own identities and, ideally, healthy self-esteem.
3. *Emotional influences:* Adolescents start to develop the ability to understand and control their emotions. They begin to comprehend relationships in a mature way and think things through from different perspectives. Yet they remain neither child nor adult.
4. *Social influences:* Adolescents tend to focus all their interest on peers and begin to develop romantic relationships. They seek more privacy from family members and want their own identities. They begin to acquire rights: to drive, to earn money, to vote, and so on. Along with these rights come added responsibilities: home obligations, academic expectations, assistance to younger siblings, contributions to home finances.

Tweens

Tweens are a newly identified group of children between ages 8 and 11 years who are entering the adolescent stage of development. Advertisers named this group of children and now target specific clothing and personal items to this market. Technology plays a significant part in enhancing this effort. Some educators and parents fear that this will lead to exposure to sexual experiences before some children are ready for them. Of course, most parents prefer that their children remain children as long as possible.

SEXUAL HEALTH ISSUES TERMINOLOGY

Homosexual	A person sexually attracted to someone of the same sex.
Heterosexual	A person sexually attracted to someone of the opposite sex.
Cisgender	A person whose gender identity and expression are aligned with the gender assigned at birth.
Ally	A member of the majority or dominant group who works to end oppression by supporting the oppressed population.
Lesbian	A female attracted sexually to another female.
Gay	A sexual orientation and/or identity of a person who is emotionally and sexually attracted to some members of the same sex. Gay can refer to both males and females or can be used as an umbrella term to refer to all lesbian, gay, and bisexual people, but some prefer the more inclusive term LGBT.
Bisexual	A sexual orientation and/or identity of a person who is emotionally and sexually attracted to some males and some females.
Transvestite	A person, typically a man, who derives pleasure from dressing as a woman.
Transgender	A person whose sense of personal identity and gender does not correspond with the birth sex.

SEXUAL HEALTH ISSUES

Sexual Orientation

Sexuality is part of the normal development of a person's identity. Adolescents frequently are fearful about their gender identity. This fear is warranted because of continuing discrimination against homosexual, bisexual, and transgender people.

Fast Facts

Sexuality can be thought of as occurring on a continuum with heterosexuality at one end and homosexuality at the other. All people are at different points on that continuum.

(*continued*)

(continued)

Clinical Snapshot

Matthew is a frail, gentle ninth grader who is frequently tormented by groups of his peers. Other students call Matthew names and harass him in the hallways. In an anonymous question box, Matthew asks the school nurse, Lisa, how he will know if he is gay.

One response might be to explain that sexuality is not a choice but a combination of genetic, hormonal, and environmental factors. Explain that there is no way that you or anyone else can tell if Matthew is gay at this age, but when he is older, it will be clearer. Assure him that he is perfect just the way he is. For now, if the subject of homosexuality, or any other topic, is really troubling him, you can arrange for Matthew to talk privately with a counselor about his feelings.

Risky Behaviors

Young adolescents have not mastered the ability to think in the long term, so they tend to be involved with behaviors that can cause immediate and long-term harm. Drinking, driving, and drug use are significant concerns during adolescence.

Teen Parenting

In recent years, there has been progress in reducing the number of teen pregnancies; however, a significant number of teens still become pregnant. This is a crisis for the adolescent mother and father and their families. Many teens choose to abort, but many others carry and keep their babies while remaining in school. Children rarely make good parents, and a baby born to teen parents will likely suffer despite the best intentions of the parents.

Sexually Transmitted Infections

The great majority of those who contract sexually transmitted infections (STIs) are younger than 25 years of age. In addition, adolescents are at high risk for reinfection because they frequently do not notify partners or seek prompt treatment. Despite the availability of drug therapy, HIV infection carries a death threat. Chlamydia, gonorrhea, and pelvic inflammatory disease are the most common STIs diagnosed among adolescents.

Fast Facts

Sexuality is an area where discretion is a priority. Do not gossip with colleagues. Make sure files are secure, and document only what you must according to district policy. We carry a tremendous responsibility for students who have mental health and sexuality issues and are just a little different. Watch the quiet ones. No one hears their voices until it is too late.

Clinical Snapshot

Amanda is a newly enrolled ninth grader. She appears depressed, isolates herself, and refuses overtures from you and her peers to participate in school functions. School nurse Lisa notices that Amanda wears long sleeves even in warm weather and is concerned she might be cutting. Lisa speaks with her and asks her if she has ever considered hurting herself. Lisa asks Amanda if she can see her arms and will refer immediately for psychiatric evaluation if scars are seen or she expresses suicidal thoughts. Lisa will continue to invite her to join the school health club or find tasks for Amanda to do in her office. Lisa will gradually help Amanda integrate into the school community while affording her a warm place to visit and find acceptance.

ROLE OF SCHOOL NURSES IN ADOLESCENT SEXUALITY

- Continue to listen and be approachable to all students.
- Empower students with education to help them make appropriate decisions.
- Remain connected to the school and community.
- Try to involve all students in some group activity.
- Permit use of appropriate bathrooms.
- Provide support within the school, especially if it is lacking at home.
- When planning to intervene, allow the adolescent to be part of the plan.
- Appreciate the importance of each student's problem, whether it is a breakup with a boyfriend or girlfriend, difficulties with peers, teasing, bullying, and so on.
- Identify any lost, unhappy children, and provide them with support.

- Check the curriculum and make sure sex education includes information about abstinence, the use of condoms, teen parenting, gender identity, and the prevention of STDs.

References

American Academy of Child and Adolescent Psychiatry. (2004). *Facts for families: Normal adolescent development.* Retrieved from www.actforyouth.net/resources/rf/rf_stages_0504.cfm

Edmonds, M. (2010). *Are teenage brains really different from adult brains?* Retrieved from http://science.howstuffworks.com/life/inside-the-mind/human-brain/teenage-brain1.htm

Garber, B. D. (2010). *Developmental psychology for family law professionals.* New York: Springer Publishing Company.

Scudder, L. E. (2006). Pediatric growth and development. In S. M. Nettina (Ed.), *Lippincott's manual of nursing practice* (8th ed.). Philadelphia, PA: Lippincott Williams & Wilkins.

Selekman, J. (Ed.). (2013). *School nursing: A comprehensive text* (pp. 2–14, 64, 1216–1243, 257–281, 407–435, 943–959, 970–997, 1135–1136). Philadelphia, PA: F.A. Davis.

16

Mental Health

School nurses know very well that the great majority of visits to the health office involve some type of emotional problem. Seldom will a motivated, happy child leave his or her classroom, whereas the needy child will want to see the nurse every day.

It is perfectly normal for children to experience a variety of emotional issues. This is part of their anticipated development and maturation. Children become anxious about school issues or have transient periods of depression much as adults do. However, when symptoms persist, they must be recognized and addressed appropriately. The child will need to rely on a system of supportive adults. You can be one of these important people.

In this chapter, you will learn:

1. The definition of *mental health*
2. The prevalence of mental illness in today's youth
3. The causes of mental illness
4. Types of mental disorders and issues affecting the school-age child
5. Strategies the school nurse can use to help identify adolescents experiencing mental health issues

DEFINITION OF MENTAL HEALTH

According to the World Health Organization (2014), *mental health* is best defined as a state of well-being in which every individual realizes his or her own potential, can cope with the normal stresses of life, can work productively and fruitfully, and is able to make a contribution to his or her community.

Mental health includes our emotional, psychological, and social well-being. It affects how we think, feel, and act. It also determines how we handle stress, relate to others, and make health choices. Mental health is important at every stage of life, from childhood and adolescence through adulthood.

Poor Mental Health Versus Mental Illness

Poor mental health and mental illness are not the same. A person can experience poor mental health yet not have a diagnosed mental illness. Those who suffer with mental illness have periods of mental health (Centers for Disease Control and Prevention [CDC], n.d.).

Mental health can and often does change. When the demands experienced by individuals exceed their resources and coping abilities, their mental health will be compromised. For example, the student who is new to the school or has unrest at home may have mental health issues. The deciding factor will be the support he or she receives. School personnel will be vital in this child's life (CDC, n.d.).

PREVALENCE OF MENTAL HEALTH ISSUES IN TODAY'S YOUTH

The statistics are frightening. According to the CDC (n.d.), attention deficit hyperactivity disorder (ADHD), behavior problems, anxiety, and depression are the most commonly diagnosed mental disorders in children:

- 9.4% of children aged 2 to 17 years (approximately 6.1 million) have received an ADHD diagnosis.
- 7.4% of children aged 3 to 17 years (approximately 4.5 million) have a diagnosed behavior problem.
- 7.1% of children aged 3 to 17 years (approximately 4.4 million) have diagnosed anxiety.
- 3.2% of children aged 3 to 17 years (approximately 1.9 million) have diagnosed depression.

CAUSES OF MENTAL ILLNESS

Most experts agree that there is no single cause for mental illness. However, we do recognize contributing factors that will increase the likelihood of a child experiencing mental illness.

1. Traumatic early childhood: Emotional, physical, or sexual abuse
2. Familial history of mental illness

3. Biological factors: Chemical imbalances in the brain
4. Substance abuse: Drugs, alcohol
5. Few social contacts, feelings of loneliness

CONTRIBUTING FACTORS

Transient Lifestyles

Children who move frequently have difficulty establishing roots and maintaining friendships. This often means they are not physically close to their extended families. They frequently do not fit in.

Adolescence

This period of time involves tremendous hormonal changes and may contribute to emotional outbursts, anxiety, and/or depression.

Need for Autonomy

Adolescents are seeking autonomy from their families, so peer involvement is essential.

Sexual Identity

Frequently children uncertain about their sexual orientation are bullied and ridiculed. This will lead to isolation and depression.

Substance Abuse

Drug or alcohol experimentation is common and can lead to addiction.

Fast Facts

Seldom will a child enter your office and tell you "I am sad and need to talk to you." Frequently, they do not understand what is wrong themselves.

Clinical Snapshot

Sixth grader Mary Ellen visits the nurse every day. Her usual complaint is an upset stomach. School nurse Emma assesses her each visit, allows her to rest, and has her return to class. Emma knows that Mary Ellen is new this year but anticipated by now she would have made some friends and found a comfortable place in the school.

(continued)

(continued)

Eventually, Emma speaks with Mary Ellen's teacher and learns that Mary Ellen has been excluded from the other girls in the class. A conference with the parents reveals that she is also being bullied. Administration is immediately informed, and guidance became involved. Emma is told she can pick one other student to help in the health office at lunchtime while investigation takes place.

MENTAL HEALTH DISORDERS AND ISSUES

The following issues are some of the mental illnesses seen in the school-age child. If unrecognized or left untreated, they can lead to school failure and tremendous suffering for the student and his or her family. It is *not* the responsibility of the school nurse to diagnose these disorders. Rather, the nurse's role is to understand their prevalence in children, observe for early signs and symptoms, be an available refuge for the student, and make referrals immediately when necessary. Frequently, following a referral, counseling will be recommended, medication will be prescribed, or both will be included.

Disruptive Disorders

Some children have more difficulty than others following directions and rules set forth in school. These disorders include the following.

Attention Deficit Hyperactivity Disorder

Signs and symptoms include:

- Difficulty completing tasks
- Easily distracted
- Disorganized
- Prone to making mistakes

Oppositional Defiant Disorder

Signs and symptoms include:

- Defiance
- Disobedience
- Hostility

Conduct Disorder

Signs and symptoms include:

- Aggressiveness

- Bullying
- Cruelty to people or animals
- Early substance abuse

Isolation

Belonging to a group and community is a fundamental need of all people. A student who frequently moves or is not accepted by peers must be closely observed. Signs and symptoms of isolation include:

- Refusal to participate in group activities
- Sudden, dramatic change in appearance
- Talk of suicide
- Talk or evidence of self-harm
- Peers expressing concern

Anxiety

Anxiety is a manifestation of stress and fear that has no clear cause. Signs and symptoms include:

- Difficulty breathing
- Nausea
- Tachycardia
- Persistent negative thoughts
- Fears that interfere with activities

Eating Disorders

Adolescents may become obsessed with looking thin to such an extreme that they become ill. The two most common eating disorders are bulimia nervosa and anorexia nervosa.

Bulimia Nervosa

Signs and symptoms of bulimia include:

- Binging: Eating a large amount of food in a short period of time
- Purging: Forcing oneself to vomit

Anorexia Nervosa

Signs and symptoms of anorexia include:

- Severe dieting
- Excessive exercise
- Abuse of laxatives

Obsessive-Compulsive Disorders

Persons with these disorders experience repetitive, unwanted thoughts that become uncontrollable, repetitive behaviors. Signs and symptoms include:

- Fear of germs
- Fear of things being out of order
- Repetitive counting, tapping, words, or phrases

Phobias

Phobias are excessive, unreasonable fears in response to objects or events. They are usually triggered by some event. Signs and symptoms of phobias include:

- Overwhelming anxiety or panic
- A need to escape
- Knowledge of overreaction but powerless to control self

Mood Disorders (Affective Disorders)

Everyone is capable of experiencing a wide range of moods, and irritability is common. Mood disorders are diagnosed when extremes of mood or irritability interfere with a student's ability to perform the activities of daily life. Signs and symptoms include:

- Depression
- Excessive fatigue
- Loss of appetite

Psychosis

Psychosis describes a mental health illness when the individual has lost some contact with reality, resulting in severe disruption in thinking and behavior. Psychosis may be present in schizophrenia and bipolar disorder (manic depression). Signs and symptoms include:

- Early change in behavior, thinking, emotions, and perception
- Trouble discerning dreams from reality
- Vivid and bizarre thoughts and ideas
- Problems in making and keeping friends

Suicide

Suicide is rare in early adolescence but becomes more common in later stages of adolescence. It remains a hidden problem and is the third leading cause of death among adolescents aged 10 to 19 years. Signs and symptoms of suicidal potential include:

- Familial history of suicide or violence
- Previous attempt
- Depression

Self-Injury Disorders

Adolescents may experience such extreme internal pain or anger that they attempt to harm themselves by cutting or undergoing excessive tattooing. Signs and symptoms of self-injury include:

- Fresh, unexplained cuts or bruises
- Wearing long sleeves in very warm weather
- Emotional instability

Healthy People 2020 Objective:
Mental Health and Mental Disorders, 4.1:
Reduce the proportion of adolescents aged 12 to 17 years who experience major depressive episodes (MDEs) from 8.3% in 2008 to 7.4%.

ROLE OF THE SCHOOL NURSE IN MENTAL HEALTH ISSUES

- Know your students. Be alert for those who might be at risk to harm themselves.
- Continue to listen and be approachable to all students.
- Remain nonjudgmental.
- Empower students with education to help them make appropriate decisions.
- Be mindful of the need for every child to have strong protective factors: Good self-esteem, feeling of self-control, good social support, positive health practices, closeness to good adult role models.
- Identify any lost, unhappy children, and provide them with support.
- Remain connected to the school and community.
- Try to involve all students in some group activity.
- Provide support within the school, especially if it is lacking at home.
- When planning to intervene, allow the adolescent to be part of the plan.
- Appreciate the importance of each student's problem, whether it is a breakup with a boyfriend or girlfriend, difficulties with peers, teasing, bullying, and so on.
- Know when to refer for evaluation. You are not a therapist.

References

Centers for Disease Control and Prevention. (n.d.). *Mental health*. Retrieved from https://www.cdc.gov/mentalhealth/learn/index.htm

World Health Organization. (2014). *Mental health: Strengthening our response* (Fact Sheet No 220). Retrieved from http://www.who.int/mediacentre/factsheets/fs220/en/

17

Drug Use

The United States' longest, yet to be won, war is the "war on drugs." We have sent millions of Americans to jail, increased penalties for offenders, seen thousands die of drug overdoses, and hopelessly beg our children to "just say no."

Different drugs become popular with different generations, and the problem persists year after year, decade after decade, and generation after generation. Today, illegal drugs are available as ever and remain even more deadly. Most feel this is one war we will never win.

As school nurses, we recognize this serious concern and sometimes wonder if we are better off today than we were decades ago. The recent legalization of marijuana in several states and the District of Columbia has also led to a more tolerant political view on recreational drug use. Medical use of marijuana in schools is becoming more acceptable, and this will definitely have an impact on our practice.

In this chapter, we explore the history of drug use over the centuries and take a fresh look at where we are today and the challenges before us.

Note that, in this chapter, information relevant to students also applies to staff members. Regarding substance abuse, the school nurse is the teacher, and the needs of both adults and students are the same in terms of requiring early detection, treatment, and support.

Confidentiality is crucial for all, although the legal parameters are different for minor children.

In this chapter, you will learn:

1. The definition of *drug abuse*
2. History of illegal drug use in the United States
3. Drugs classified as opioids and overdose treatment with naloxone
4. The definition of *vaping* and use of e-cigarettes
5. Risk factors and protective factors that influence students
6. The levels of school and district drug education programs
7. How to develop a prevention plan for those at risk, and strategies to help those who are already dependent

DEFINITION

Drug Use and Abuse

A drug is a chemical substance that affects the way the body or mind functions. Drugs can treat diseases, promote health, or make a person ill, depending on how they are used. The inappropriate use of any drug, under any circumstances, is considered abuse.

Fast Facts

Drugs that can cause dependence are restricted by age (e.g., tobacco and alcohol), availability (e.g., prescription pain medication), or laws (e.g., marijuana and cocaine).

Clinical Snapshot

School nurse Helen is becoming increasingly concerned about a senior student, David. His attendance is poor, and he is a social isolate. After attending a class on addiction, he reveals that his parents have a variety of common ailments and, therefore, they have a medicine cabinet stocked with numerous medications for their use. David began abusing drugs at age 16 following an orthopedic injury, with his parents completely unaware that he was slowly, systematically helping himself to their medications and becoming increasingly addicted.

HISTORY OF ILLEGAL DRUG USE IN THE UNITED STATES

Opium is considered the first drug to be used and adapted for illegal use. Opium is developed from the unripe poppy see pod. The milky fluid is taken from the unripe seed pod, it is dried, and the resin is sold as opium.

From opium, alkaloids such as morphine, codeine, and heroin were developed. Initially, these products were believed to be less addictive than opium. The development of the syringe and ability to inject directly into the bloodstream further enhanced the effects of these narcotics.

The United States, as many countries, has a long history of drug use/abuse (see Table 17.1). The specific drug abused in any generation changes, but it is not a new problem by any means. State laws are being passed influencing federal laws. When the state law allows a drug for medicinal purposes, the federal laws are secondary.

Table 17.1

Historical Timeline of Illegal Drug Use in the United States

Before 19th century	Substance abuse was primarily related to plant-produced products and alcohol. These substances were dangerous and addictive, but at that time, we lacked knowledge of addiction.
1803	From opium, alkaloids such as morphine, codeine, cocaine, and heroin were developed. These products were manufactured in the lab. The development of the syringe also enhanced the effects of these narcotics. Drugs were not regulated and were easy to obtain.
1914	The Harrison Act caused development of positive changes in drug treatment. Narcotics were only available with a prescription.
1936	Federal Bureau of Narcotics was organized and took a stand against drug abuse.
1960	Drugs were used for recreational purposes: marijuana, LSD, cocaine, heroin, hallucinogens.
1965	Amphetamines (speed) became popular with young adults.
1980	Hallucinogens and cocaine were used in social settings. Schools adopted policies for students suspected of drug use.
1985	Crack cocaine, a freebase form of cocaine made by cooking cocaine powder, water, and baking soda until it forms a solid that can be broken down and sold in pieces or "rocks," was developed. Crack is highly addictive.
1990	Crystal methamphetamine was in use. Ice increased in heroin use—smoked and snorted.
2016	Opioids become major threat. Narcan was developed to reverse reaction.
2017	Some states legalize recreational use of marijuana. Physician-directed medical use is permitted in some schools for specific conditions.

Schools attempt to educate, yet we continue to contribute to the history of drug abuse.

OPIODS AND OVERDOSE TREATMENT WITH NALOXONE

Opioids

Drugs classified as opioid act by binding to opioid receptors in the brain and blocking pain receptors. Some opioids are commonly prescribed by physicians. They are prescribed under names such as oxycodone (OxyContin), hydrocondone (Vicodin), codeine, and morphine. Heroin and fentanyl are illegal.

We now know that regular use of any opioid can lead to dependence and addiction, regardless of whether the drug has been prescribed by a physician or purchased illegally. A 16-year-old prescribed any opioid following wisdom teeth extraction or athletic injury can unknowingly become dependent/addicted. Opioids, both prescription and illicit, are the main driver of drug overdose deaths.

Opioid overdose was involved in 47,600 deaths in 2017. These numbers represent an increase five times higher in 2016 than 1999. This accounts for 115 deaths per day! (Centers for Disease Control and Prevention [CDC], 2017)

Naloxone (Narcan)

There has been little progress in drug prevention programs. Naloxone (Narcan), an overdose-reversal drug, is now a required stock drug kept in many schools. It is the first-known drug in death-prevention treatment.

In 2016, we saw 32,000 deaths due to motor vehicle crashes (CDC, 2016). Consider today's large number of effective preventive measures now required of car manufacturers (seat belts, air bags, rear camera, etc.). Sadly, with a much greater number of deaths due to drug use, prevention has not been effective.

Attempts have been made to limit opioid prescriptions to 7 as opposed to 30 days. Physicians have been encouraged to caution patients about the use/abuse of opioids, and locations where unused prescription drugs can be safely discarded are prevalent.

Obviously, drug abuse and the concerns of today are quite different from those of the past. More over-the-counter and prescription drugs are being used by younger children (CDC, 2010). Gateway drugs such as alcohol and tobacco are being tried by children as young as 9 or 10 years of age. At such early ages, addiction is more likely and costly in terms of both monetary funds and academic performance. The emotional toll is even more devastating. The undeveloped brain of the adolescent is highly susceptible to addiction. Large-scale national and state programs have not made the hoped-for impact of changing behavior.

Healthy People 2020 Objectives
Substance Abuse, 19.5
Reduce the past-year nonmedical use of any psychotherapeutic drug (including pain relievers, tranquilizers, stimulants, and sedatives) by person aged 12 years and older from 6.1% in 2008 to 5.5%.

Vaping and E-Cigarettes

Tobacco use has long been linked to lung cancer, other respiratory conditions, and cardiac diseases. School nurses and health professionals recognize that tobacco is a gateway drug frequently leading to drug abuse.

Vaping means to inhale vapor through the mouth from an electronic device that heats up and vaporizes a liquid or solid.

Since around 2011 the use of e-cigarettes has grown in alarming rates among teens. E-cigarettes are electronic nicotine delivery systems in a battery-operated device. It delivers a mixture of nicotine, flavoring, and other chemicals in a vapor that is inhaled directly into the lungs.

We do not know much about the long-term effects of e-cigarettes and vaping, but with no Food and Drug Administration (FDA) oversight, there is cause for school nurses to be concerned as with all nicotine products.

Risk Factors

- Aggressive behavior at a young age
- Unrest within the family
- Family members or close peers who abuse drugs
- Low income levels
- Mentally challenged
- Drug availability
- Low self-esteem
- Social ineptness

Students who are less likely to abuse drugs have what are called protective factors.

Protective Factors

- Stable family life
- Adequate income level
- Community and school support
- Good social skills

- Disciplined lifestyle
- Confidence
- Resistance skills
- Academic achievement

THE GOAL

According to the National Institute on Drug Abuse (2010, p. 7), the goal of preventive programs for students with risk factors is to change the balance of risk factors and protective factors so that students are more protected than at risk.

TIMES OF GREATEST RISK

It is especially important to support high-risk students during times of major life transitions. The need to be included and to belong is important to all of us, but for these students, during these times, it is crucial. These times include the following:

- Parents' divorcing
- Changing schools
- Moving
- A sudden illness of the student or a family member
- A stressful environment (e.g., bullying)

TYPES OF PROGRAMS

To best meet the drug education needs of all students, every school and district should have three levels of programs.

Level One: Preventive (For All Students)

Schools today must teach health education as part of the required content areas for learning. The curriculum, learning objectives, and lesson plans are written by the classroom teacher to address the specific drug education needs of the learners. The health teacher must first understand what drugs are commonly used by the students in his or her classes and focus on these.

Level Two: Preventive (For High-Risk Students)

Know your students. Recognize the students at risk and the times that create extreme stress in their lives, and be available. Approach these students, acknowledge the difficult time they are having, and ask that they let you know if they need help. Check resources within the school system. If necessary, offer to investigate available community programs that work with high-risk students and provide prevention strategies to avoid experimenting with drugs or alcohol and halt the progression into drug dependence. This is the area in which much can be done and the school nurse can be most effective.

Level Three: Intervention (For Those Already Drug Dependent)

Once a person is diagnosed and involved in a treatment plan, the school nurse can be invaluable in offering support to the student and his or her family once they return to school. Know what the student's follow-up plan entails, and seek to be part of it.

Fast Facts

Parental attitudes toward drug use can be a major obstacle. Be aware of what is acceptable at home before you attempt to work with the student. You may need to begin by educating the parents.

Clinical Snapshot

David Johnson is 17, the youngest of three children. His older siblings attended prestigious universities and are successful and productive citizens The liquor cabinet in his home has always been left open and available to him, as it was to his brothers. His parents expect that he will drink with his friends, both at home and away from home. They ask only that he not drive while intoxicated. The Johnsons permit other underaged children to drink in their home as well and are in denial that any harm could come from this arrangement. Helen is aware that some of this drinking is occurring at lunchtime and informs the parents that she will follow the school policy on reporting suspicion of alcohol use. She works with her school's parent group to conduct educational programs in an attempt to change attitudes toward underage drinking.

PREVENTIVE APPROACH FOR ALL STUDENTS

A preventive approach is effective for the vast number of students. Teachers are highly qualified to provide factual, necessary information and guide students to make prudent choices.

Role of School Nurses in the Preventive Approach for All Students

- Be a role model for healthful habits.
- Question the student returning to school following injury or surgery concerning what pain medication he or she is taking.
- Stay current with information on drug use in your school and community.
- Check on what is presently taught in the classrooms.
- Help write the health curriculum.
- Make time in your busy schedule to teach, both in the classroom and one-on-one.
- Partner with community organizations such as the parent–teacher association (PTA) and the police (Drug Abuse Resistance Education) to offer special learning opportunities for students.
- Know your district's policies and procedures for suspected drug abuse. If you disagree, question and seek change *before* any incidents occur.

PREVENTIVE PROGRAMS FOR HIGH-RISK STUDENTS

A health education program such as that outlined earlier is sufficient for most students. However, the greatest concern is for students with risk factors for substance use. Students with one or more of the following characteristics, such as frequent moves, parental divorce, and being bullied, are more likely than others to abuse drugs.

Role of School Nurses in Preventive Programs for High-Risk Students

- Be available to everyone. Keep your door open and the atmosphere in your office warm and inviting.
- Do not be afraid to befriend the student, families, and staff members you feel are at risk.
- Build a support system within the school (you, classroom teachers, peer advisors, guidance counselors, administrators).
- Develop a plan:
    - Identify the risk factor(s).
    - Set goals for students.
    - Provide a "safe" place for students to go. Allow them access to your office whenever the need arises without them having to state a specific illness.
    - Analyze students' day(s), and remove or relieve stressful factors (e.g., an uncompromising teacher or peer bullying).
- Evaluate students' progress as needed, and revise your plans accordingly.
- Reassure students that you sincerely care about their well-being and that each of them is an important part of the school.

INTERVENTION PROGRAMS FOR THOSE ALREADY DRUG DEPENDENT

Once a student has been identified as having a drug problem, the school district's policies and procedures will dictate when the student is to be excluded, how the student is to be monitored during the recovery period, and when the student can be readmitted to school. Follow-up will also be addressed, and the school nurse will continue to be involved. This is the time when you need to be more diligent than ever. You do not want this child to be truant or to drop out of school. Treat the addicted child's absence with the same concern you demonstrate for any child with a chronic illness. You can make the difference in this student's recovery.

Fast Facts

Do not attempt to counsel a student on your own. This is not your role. Work with the school's team of professionals, and implement the school's policies and procedures.

Clinical Snapshot

Helen reports her concerns to the guidance and drug counselors at school. Together they meet with David's parents to explain what they suspect.

Parents will frequently confide in you, seeking your approval and support. Maintain professional boundaries, listen, and encourage them to seek appropriate services, in or out of school.

WHY SCHOOLS HAVE SO MUCH RESPONSIBILITY IN THIS AREA

The reader might now be thinking, Why does the school (and I, myself, in particular) have such a great responsibility? What about the parents, family members, other teachers, the community, and religious institutions? Consider the following facts:

- Children must attend school for approximately 5 hours a day, which is far more time than many of them spend with their parents. Students are a captive audience for us.
- As with most health topics, drug education *should* be taught at home. The sad fact is, however, that it is not. We must pick up that slack.

- Parents are sometimes not the best role models. *You are.* You made that decision when you chose a health profession, and you renewed that commitment when you started your school nursing career.

As far as the health needs of your students are concerned, as always, you know what is best.

Role of School Nurses in Intervention Programs for Those Already Drug Dependent

- Encourage the student to return to school as soon as possible.
- Welcome the student back, set aside time in your day to see the student, and help him or her to readjust and catch up on missed schoolwork.
- Keep in touch with the home, family physician, and any outside agency involved.
- Remain discrete. Know where to document drug-related information, and do not violate your district's policy on confidentiality.

References

Centers for Disease Control and Prevention. (2010). *Prescription drug use continues to increase: U.S. prescription drug data for 2007–2008*. Retrieved from https://www.cdc.gov/nchs/products/databriefs/db42.htm

Centers for Disease Control and Prevention. (2016). *Motor vehicle crash deaths*. Retrieved from https://www.cdc.gov/vitalsigns/motor-vehicle-safety/index.html

Centers for Disease Control and Prevention. (2017). *Drug overdose deaths*. Retrieved from https://www.cdc.gov/drugoverdose/data/statedeaths.html

National Institute on Drug Abuse. (2010). *Preventing drug abuse among children and adults: Risk factors and protective factors*. Publication no. 10-7583. Retrieved from http://www.nida.nih.gov/prevention/risk.html

18

Bullies and Their Victims

Comforting a child who has just been bullied is one of the most painful parts of a school nurse's job. Comforting parents who are dealing with cruelty inflicted on their child is even worse. But hearing about a child who has been tormented for months that you were unaware of is the worst possible situation you could find yourself in.

Sadly, this is far too often the case. This chapter hopefully creates a greater awareness of the scope of this problem. It is placed in the part of the book that deals with the marginalized child. These children on the margins or fringes of society are the most susceptible and the most vulnerable to the bully. This is the child who is different and does not fit in. The child might have cultural differences, special needs, morbid obesity, mental illness, gender identity issues, abusive relationships, or be addicted to drugs.

You have responsibilities to the entire school, but these are the students who need you most. Consider the marginalized students your class. You must go above and beyond to help them find their place and meet academic as well as social success.

In this chapter, you will learn:

1. Definitions of bullying, harassment, and intimidation
2. Types of bullying
3. Scope of the problem
4. The effects of bullying

5. Possible school interventions
6. Actions for the school nurse

DEFINITIONS

Bullying

Bullying is unwanted, repeated, aggressive behavior among school-age children that involves a real or perceived power imbalance.

Bullying remains the most frequently reported disciplinary problem in schools. According to information provided in "Indicators of School Crime and Safety: 2016" (National Center for Education Statistics, 2017). In 2015, among students ages 12 to 18, 21% of students reported being bullied at school during the school year. In 2015, about 15% of U.S. fourth graders reported experiencing bullying at least once a month. Because bullying is so commonplace and ranges in severity, its impact is very often overlooked.

Healthy People 2020 Objectives:
Injury and Violence Prevention, 35:
Reduce the percentage of students in grades 9 through 12 who reported that they were bullied on school property in the previous 12 months from 17.97% in 2009 to 17.9%.

Harassment

Harassment means that a person is annoyed persistently. The verbal or physical conduct has created an unpleasant, even hostile, environment.

Bullying and harassment are similar as they are both about:

- Power and control
- Actions that hurt or harm another person physically or emotionally
- An imbalance of power between the target and the individual demonstrating the negative behavior
- The target having difficulty stopping the action directed at him or her

The distinction between bullying and harassment is that when the bullying behavior directed at the target is also based on race, color, religion, sex, age, disability, or national origin, that behavior is then defined as harassment.

Healthy People 2020 Objectives:
Adolescent Health, 9:
Increase the proportion of middle and high schools that prohibit harassment based on a student's sexual orientation or gender identity from 88.2% to 92.2%.

Intimidation

Intimidation is to frighten someone and cause the person to be fearful. This usually involves threats of physical or emotional harm. The person intimidating is perceived as bigger and more powerful than the victim.

TYPES OF BULLYING

Verbal

Verbal is saying or writing mean things. It includes:

- Teasing
- Name-calling
- Inappropriate sexual comments
- Taunting
- Threatening to inflict harm

Social

Social bullying is referred to as *relational bullying*. It involves hurting someone's reputation or relationships. Social bullying includes:

- Excluding someone intentionally
- Telling others to not be friends with someone
- Spreading rumors
- Embarrassing someone in public

Physical

Physical bullying involves hurting a person's body or possessions. It includes:

- Hitting/slapping/punching/pinching/kicking
- Spitting

- Tripping/pushing
- Taking or breaking someone's possessions
- Making mean or rude hand gestures

Cyber

Cyberbullying is the use of electronic devices and media such as cell phones, email, instant messaging, chat rooms, or social networking to threaten, harass, or intimidate someone. It is blamed for much of the bullying today. Bear in mind that the school still has a responsibility to act even if the bullying is done from a home computer or personal device. It includes:

- Sharing an embarrassing photo or video without permission
- Spreading rumors
- Pretending to be another person
- Threatening another person
- Sending provocative insults
- Gay bashing
- Infecting another's computer

SCOPE OF PROBLEM

In 2016, the National Center for Educational Statistics (NCES, 2017) reported that one out of every five (20.8%) students reported being bullied. Bullying occurs most frequently where there is less adult supervision.

- Hallway or stairwell (42%)
- Cafeteria (22%)
- Outside on school grounds (19%)
- School bus (10%)
- Bathroom or locker room (9%)

Common Causes of Bullying

The reasons for being bullied reported most often by students include:

- Physical appearance (obesity, large or small stature)
- Race
- Gender
- Disability
- Religion
- Sexual orientation
- Intelligence

THE EFFECTS OF BULLYING

It is now recognized that the harmful effects of bullying can manifest itself in a variety of physical and psychological ways. These effects can continue into adulthood.

It is not uncommon to hear of sleep disturbances that impact the student's ability to function in a normal school or social setting.

Depression is common, and many refuse to attend school. Gastrointestinal problems are common, as are headaches.

These are the children most likely to contemplate or actually attempt suicide.

Fast Facts

The school is legally responsible for the student's safety while on school property and going to and from school. Be alert for possible altercations during the school day that could escalate into violent acts after school.

Clinical Snapshot

It was after 4:00 p.m. when school nurse Patricia was signing out for the weekend in the now-empty main office. A mother entered crying with her son, David, who was also crying. The sixth grader had severe swelling on his right cheek and was bleeding through his pants from both knees.

David's mother demanded to see an administrator. She stated that following an altercation in class, two boys followed her son, David, home and repeatedly punched and kicked him. She claimed that these same boys have been intimidating her son for weeks.

Both parents had come in and spoken to the classroom teacher earlier that week and gotten reassurance that this intimidation would cease. Today, David's mother alleged that the teacher was aware of the altercation, did *not* intervene, and allowed her son to leave school, knowing there were threats to him, thus permitting the beating to take place.

Patricia checked the sign-out book and saw that the teacher was long gone, as was everyone else, including administration. She then tried to reach the principal by phone and was not successful.

Patricia invited David and his mom back to her office, rendered first aid, and explained that all had left but she would help as best

(*continued*)

(continued)

as she could. Taking careful notes, Patricia sensed that this situation could continue to escalate over the weekend.

Patricia contacted the parents of both boys and insisted they immediately come to school. Both sets of parents were angry and upset with their sons and promised no further incidents would happen. With all the parents' knowledge, Patricia reported the incident to the police department. The police agreed to intervene if any further incidents took place over the weekend.

What Can Be Done?

Many states have initiated antibullying laws specific to the needs of school-age children. These laws go a long way in establishing schools as a safe refuge for children.

School-based bully prevention programs decrease bullying by up to 25% (McCallion & Feder, 2013). More than half of bully situations (57%) stop when a peer intervenes on behalf of the student being bullied (Hawkins, Pepler, & Craig, 2001). This appears to be one solution that warrants continued implementations in all schools.

The most important action we can take as school nurses is to assume *every* accusation of harassment, intimidation, and bullying as a potentially serious threat to a child. Far too often, this is recognized in hindsight after permanent physical or emotional damage has been done to the child.

SCHOOL INITIATIVES TO PREVENT BULLYING

1. Provide increased supervision in areas such as cafeteria, restrooms, hallways, school bus, and locker rooms.
2. Have in place clear policies to deal with, report, and follow up with bullying allegations. Make sure they are adhered to.
3. If your school does not have a bullying policy, work with nursing colleagues and administration to develop one.
4. Stagger recess and lunchtimes so fewer children are supervised at one time.
5. Consider setting up closed-circuit cameras in hallways, stairwells, and/or cafeterias.
6. Provide teachers with classroom management strategies to deal with bullying.

7. If age appropriate, allow a peer advisory council to support students who are bullied.
8. Reward positive behavior.
9. Involve parents, students, teachers, and administrators in planning and executing plans for a bully-free school.
10. Support strict disciplinary measures for threats and acts of aggression.

ROLE OF SCHOOL NURSES IN DEALING WITH BULLYING

1. Offer opportunities for class discussions related to bullying.
2. Involve students in establishing rules against bullying and steps they can take if they see any incident of bullying, harassment, or intimidation.
3. Assign projects that will require students to work together in small groups.
4. Immediately deal with acts of bullying.
5. Speak to the bully in private. Do not confront with others present.
6. Do not mediate a bullying situation unless forced to do so.
7. Refer to an administrator or counselor, and follow up to make sure action was taken.
8. Provide your office as a safe refuge for victims as needed.
9. Insist that parents of both victim and bully be informed when problems arise.
10. Seek to resolve problems at school before going home.

References

Hawkins, D. L., Pepler, D. J., & Craig, W. M. (2001). Naturalistic observations of peer interventions in bullying. *Social Development, 10*(4), 512–527. doi:10.1111/1467-9507.00178. Retrieved from https://psycnet.apa.org/record/2001-05565-005

McCallion, G., & Feder, J. (2013). *Student Bullying: Overview of research, federal initiatives, and legal issues.* Retrieved from https://fas.org/sgp/crs/misc/R43254.pdf

National Center for Education Statistics. (2017). *Indicators of school crime and safety: 2016.* Retrieved from https://nces.ed.gov/pubs2017/2017064.pdf

19

Child Abuse

At one time, people might have thought that there was no such thing as child abuse. Prior to compulsory school attendance, many were oblivious to what was going on in homes across the country. However, as large numbers of students gathered in schools, comparisons among children became inevitable. School personnel were able to clearly identify the students who were happy and thriving in their home and school environments and those who were not. Schools today now play an important role in early detection of child abuse.

The sooner child abuse is recognized, reported, and help provided to the family, the greater the chance that the child will heal and not perpetuate the cycle.

In this chapter, you will learn:

1. Definitions of *institutional* and *noninstitutional child abuse*
2. Major aspects of the Child Abuse Prevention and Treatment Act (CAPTA)
3. Types of child abuse and neglect, along with warning signs, risk factors, and prevention strategies
4. Basic referral processes and the school's responsibility in documenting and reporting suspicions of child abuse and neglect

DEFINITIONS OF CHILD ABUSE

Broadly defined, *child abuse* is an omission of nurturing. Abuse includes much more than physical harm. In the past, when people thought of child abuse, many immediately imagined a child with visible bruises and broken bones. As distressing as this image is, there are less obvious, but equally damaging, types of child abuse that are far more common. These leave deep, long-lasting scars that have a ripple effect on families from past to present generations and generations yet to come.

One problem regarding child abuse today, as in earlier days, is how to distinguish abuse from overzealous parenting or teaching that intentionally or accidentally causes injury. There is still no consensus as to exactly what constitutes effective parental and school discipline and what constitutes abuse.

INSTITUTIONAL AND NONINSTITUTIONAL CHILD ABUSE

Child abuse can occur anywhere and anytime. The abuser can be a stranger, teacher, trusted friend, family member, priest, rabbi, scout leader, caretaker, school employee, or healthcare provider.

Institutional abuse occurs when an act of abuse takes place in a school or any formal institutional facility. The perpetrator might be a staff member, teacher, principal, older student, or custodian. Each school district has in place policies and procedures to deal with allegations of abuse by staff members and other employees.

Noninstitutional abuse occurs in homes. The perpetrator is usually a parent, relative, or someone else whom a parent has entrusted to watch the child.

Fast Facts

Each state has specific laws addressing child abuse. All states require that knowledge of alleged offenses or suspected incidences of child abuse be reported by school personnel, regardless of where these alleged offenses or incidences occurred or by whom they were committed.

Clinical Snapshot

Eight-year-old Jorge arrives in school with a lacerated lip and profuse nosebleed. Jorge states his mother hit him because he would not finish breakfast. Jorge's mom is a close friend of school nurse Margaret, and she is certain he is lying. She calls home to have Jorge's mom come and take him to be evaluated for suturing. When Jorge's mother arrives at school, she explains that he fell. Margaret accepts her word and does not refer the incident to child protective services.

(*continued*)

(*continued*)

The following week Jorge arrives at school with several teeth missing. He again states that his mother hit him. Margaret now makes the referral, angry with herself that she allowed a friendship to interfere with following proper procedure, heartsick that she permitted a child to go home to an unsafe environment, and fearful that she has left herself and her district liable for failing to report suspicion of child abuse.

Healthy People 2020 Objectives:
Injury and Violence Prevention, 38:
Reduce nonfatal maltreatment from 9.4% per 1,000 children under age 18 years in 2008 to 8.5%.

CHILD ABUSE PREVENTION AND TREATMENT ACT

The key federal legislation addressing child abuse and neglect is the CAPTA, originally enacted on January 31, 1974 (P.L. 93–247). This act has been amended several times and was last reauthorized on December 20, 2010, by the CAPTA Reauthorization Act of 2010 (P.L. 111–320). Most recently, certain provisions of the act were amended on May 29, 2015, by the Justice for Victims of Trafficking Act of 2015 (P.L. 114–122) and on July 22, 2016, by the Comprehensive Addiction and Recovery Act of 2016 (P.L. 114–198) (Child Welfare Information Gateway, 2017).

CAPTA covers all persons under 18 years of age and provides federal money to states in support of prevention, assessment, treatment, and prosecution of offenders. CAPTA defines *child abuse* as:

> at a minimum, any recent act or failure to act on the part of a parent or caretaker which results in death, serious physical or emotional harm, sexual abuse or exploitation, or an act or failure to act which presents an imminent risk of serious harm. (Child Welfare Information Gateway, 2007; EveryCRSReport.com, n.d.)

CAPTA provides federal money to all states to help implement programs that identify, treat, and prevent child abuse. To be granted this money, states must do the following:

- Indicate who are considered the reporters.
- Offer a clear definition of *maltreatment.*
- Identify the agreed-upon procedure for reporting suspected abuse and neglect.

- Indicate the agency that will receive and investigate the reports.
- Provide immunity from prosecution for good-faith reporters.
- Provide penalties for failure to report as well as for the issuing of false reports (misdemeanors punishable by fines or imprisonment, or both).
- Include additional provisions that nullify certain communication rights.
- Add additional provisions unique to the state.

CATEGORIES OF CHILD ABUSE

There are four general classifications of child abuse: physical abuse, sexual abuse, emotional abuse, and neglect. Any of these may occur separately, but they more often occur in combination. All have devastating emotional impacts on children and severely limit their ability to learn. The descriptions and lists of indicators that follow were adapted from the National Children's Advocacy Center (2010), the Child Welfare Information Gateway (2013), and the Centers for Disease Control and Prevention (CDC, 2013).

Physical Abuse

Physical abuse is reported most frequently because bruises and broken bones are visibly obvious and immediately raise suspicions. Such abuse involves physical harm or injury, which may be intentional or a result of severe discipline. Family background and cultural traditions play a role in physical abuse patterns. Some parents insist that it is their right and responsibility to use force to teach their children right from wrong. Physical abuse includes punching, beating, shaking, or hitting a victim with the hand or an object. Such victims learn to live in fear.

> *Physical indicators:* Unexplained bruises, abrasions, fractures, lacerations, or welts
>
> *Behavioral indicators:* Anxiety about going home, wariness of adults, extreme withdrawal or aggressiveness, fear of the perpetrator, frequent reports of injuries by parents, the wearing of seasonally inappropriate clothing to cover arms or legs, and self-destructive actions

Sexual Abuse

Sexual abuse includes actions by a perpetrator such as inappropriate touching of the breasts or genitals, actual penetration, incest, rape, sodomy, indecent exposure, and exploitation through prostitution or the production of pornographic materials. Sexual abuse does not necessarily involve bodily contact. A child's exposure to sexual situations or materials is also considered to be abuse.

Physical indicators: Urinary tract infections; difficulty walking or sitting; torn, stained, or bloody underclothing; pain or itching in the genital area; bruises or bleeding in the external genitalia; venereal disease; and pregnancy

Behavioral indicators: Extreme modesty; withdrawn behavior; fantasized or infantile behavior; bizarre, sophisticated, or unusual sexual behavior; poor peer relationships; delinquent or runaway behavior; reports of sexual assault; suicide attempts; and extreme weight change

Fast Facts

Sexual abuse is especially frightening because it frequently remains hidden and creates feelings of guilt and shame in the victim. Usually, the offender is someone the child knows and trusts. The child often feels responsible and may experience sexual problems as he or she gets older.

Clinical Snapshot

Jorge's mom has a live-in boyfriend whom Jorge clearly fears. You notice that Jorge frequently stops in to see you after school to delay going home. Margaret needs to ask Jorge the hard questions. Is he afraid to go home? Why does he dislike his mother's boyfriend? Has his mother's boyfriend ever tried to touch him inappropriately?

Emotional Abuse

Emotional abuse can severely damage a child's self-esteem and social development. Such abuse is usually repetitive and includes verbal insults or severe punishment. The scars are lifelong and can lead to psychiatric issues. The impact of emotional abuse can be even greater than sexual or physical abuse. Examples of emotional abuse include constant belittling, humiliating, name-calling, threatening, bullying, ignoring, and rejecting a child as punishment; limited physical contact (e.g., lack of hugging, kissing, and affection); and exposing a child to violence or abuse by others.

Physical indicators: Habit disorders such as sucking, biting, or rocking; conduct disorders such as antisocial or destructive behavior; and neurotic traits, including sleep disorders, speech disorders, and inhibition of play

Behavioral indicators: Behavior extremes, overly adaptive behavior, and attempted suicide

Neglect

Child neglect is the failure to provide for a child's basic needs. Neglect is not often reported or apparent to the casual observer. Children have a remarkable way of adapting, and they may blame themselves for a lack of nurturing from their parents. Many more children experience neglect than are either physically or sexually abused.

Areas of Child Neglect

- *Physical neglect:* Failure to provide adequate food, clothing, shelter, or supervision
- *Medical neglect:* Failure to provide needed medical care
- *Educational neglect:* Failure to provide education or to tend to the special needs of a child
- *Emotional neglect:* Failure to tend to a child's emotional needs or to provide psychological care, or permitting a child to use alcohol or drugs

Neglect is the most common form of child abuse. Many teachers will simply choose to ignore it rather than jeopardize their relationship with the parent. You will be able to help in this area better than anyone else in the school.

Physical indicators: Hunger, poor hygiene, inappropriate clothing, lack of supervision, fatigue, unattended physical problems or medical needs, and abandonment

Behavioral indicators: Begging, stealing food or other items, reluctance to leave school, falling asleep in class, substance abuse, delinquency, dropping out of school, and no known caregiver

As professional caregivers we find it difficult to fathom that some children are abused and neglected by their parents. Many parents are also tolerant of abuse that occurs in schools. Some parents even encourage teachers to use physical punishment, completely trusting the staff and believing that such punishment will benefit their children.

What is especially upsetting is that society as a whole must acknowledge being a part of creating and maintaining an atmosphere that may lead to child abuse. Poverty, transient lifestyles, single parenting, overexposure to violence in the media, and inadequate child protective service agencies all contribute to an environment that increases the likelihood of neglect and abuse. The horror of child abuse, therefore, is not a simple issue that exists only between the victim and the perpetrator. We must look at the bigger picture and the role that we play in it.

RISK FACTORS FOR CHILD ABUSE

Certain conditions or situations place students at risk for abuse. They include the following:

Poverty: All too often, adequate services are not available to poor families. When a parent is unemployed or ill, the family may have inadequate food, clothing, and overcrowded living conditions. Poor people tend to move frequently, causing further unease. In addition, most illegal immigrants are afraid to report their needs lest they be deported.

Violence in the home: It is terrifying for a child to witness violence among family members. Children suffer tremendous emotional damage when they are subjected to violence in the home.

Parental history of abuse: If either parent has been abused, it is likely that he or she will perpetuate the abuse cycle.

Lack of parenting skills: Parents who are very young, mentally unstable, or have never had good role models often do not know how to nurture their children properly.

Mental illness: If they are not diagnosed and treated, parents with mental illness may direct their anger and frustrations toward their children.

Transient lifestyle: Parents who often move from place to place may not live near other family members, and therefore, they have little or no support.

Substance abuse: Parents who are substance abusers are often child abusers as well. Their judgment is poor and inconsistent.

PREVENTION STRATEGIES

As with many other issues, prevention is the key, and education is the only way to achieve it.

Education of Staff

This can be done through yearly educational programs so that teachers and staff can recognize the signs of child abuse and neglect and understand their role in the process of prevention, detection, and referral.

Education for Students

Children need to be empowered with information to protect themselves. The best way to accomplish this is to offer a comprehensive school health curriculum focusing on prevention strategies for children.

Education for Parents

In some cases, parents need outside resources to cope with parenting in appropriate ways. Counseling services and educational programs are available, and the school nurse can facilitate parental access. Parents need to know that it is the law that all *suspected* cases of child abuse and neglect must be reported by school officials.

Fast Facts

After Margaret makes the call to Children's Protective Services, she informs the principal of her actions. Within 5 minutes the classroom teacher is in her office, complaining that she had not been informed.

Be clear as to which administrator you will share information with. Remain discreet, and keep *only* that person informed. You tend to the needs of the child; let administrators take care of staff and each other. Check your state's policy. If you believe you will be penalized for reporting a suspicion of abuse, you may not have to inform any school administrator.

Clinical Snapshot

Jorge also shares with you that his 19-year-old cousin is always trying to get him alone to kiss and touch his private parts. Margaret makes the referral and informs the principal that a representative from child protective services is coming to the school. The guidance counselor, secretaries, and custodial staff want to know what is going on. Out of respect for the child and family members, Margaret does not share this information. Instead, she refers them to the principal.

Fast Facts

Calling a child protective services agency is a difficult thing to do. Many people just do not want to get involved. Any nurse with this attitude should find a specialty other than that of school nursing. Protecting children is part of a school nurse's job, and the nurse "got involved" on the day that he or she chose school nursing.

Clinical Snapshot

Margaret checks her mailbox just before leaving school for the weekend. She finds a note from a third-grade teacher, informing her of an alleged incident of noninstitutional sexual abuse involving one of her students that was reported to the teacher that morning. The teacher asks her to look into it. The teacher, student, and building administrator have already left for the weekend. Margaret is furious with the teacher but returns to her office and makes the referral call, knowing that she has acted in the best interest of that child. Before leaving the building, Margaret calls the teacher and principal at their homes and demands to meet with them on Monday to discuss their professional responsibilities.

BASIC REFERRAL PROCESS

Most states have regulations requiring the "first person contact" to make a referral. This means that whoever speaks with a child *first* about abuse or neglect, or whoever has a strong suspicion that abuse is occurring, must report it to the proper agency themselves. You can assist reporters of abuse or neglect by providing the appropriate phone numbers and any history of the child that you are aware of, but the responsibility to call is *theirs*.

The steps in this process are as follows:

1. You or another adult has *reasonable cause* to believe that a child is being abused or neglected. If a child has a visible bruise and states, "My father hit me," then it is clear that a referral is necessary. Most cases are not as obvious. A child might be afraid to admit that a parent hurt him or her lest this anger the parent or cause the child to be removed from the home.
2. In good faith, the child protective services agency is notified. If you are uncertain whether the child was hit by the parent, you can explain that to the caseworker, who will investigate.

3. Provide the agency with the necessary information: the child's name, address, the names of any siblings, the parents' names, phone numbers, workplaces, and so on.
4. Make the call early in the day if possible. Often, an investigator will need to come to the school to speak with the child.
5. Insist on seeing identification from anyone asking to speak with the child in school, and remain present to support the child.
6. Document according to district policy.
7. Follow up on all referrals.

ROLE OF SCHOOL NURSES IN CHILD ABUSE

Preventive Strategies

- Be alert to the risk factors in a child's life.
- Recognize the early signs, symptoms, and behavioral indicators of child neglect and abuse.
- Know your district's policy on reporting child abuse.
- Arrange staff educational programs. Teach the signs and symptoms of child abuse to the entire staff: teachers, lunch aides, classroom aides, bus drivers, after-school personnel, coaches, and so on.
- Caution staff members not to place themselves in positions where they are alone with students and can be accused of child abuse.
- Develop a zero-tolerance approach for child abuse and neglect.
- Make certain that information about the individual's right to privacy and protection of his or her own body is provided to students via the health education curriculum.
- Inform all parents and staff, in writing and publicly at meetings, that the first person contact *by law* is to report all incidents of suspected child abuse.
- Accept that this part of your job is ugly, but it must be done.

Detection and Reporting Strategies

- Be available to listen and ready to ask the difficult questions.
- When speaking with a child, use objective, not leading, questioning techniques: "Tell me about that bruise" as opposed to "Who hit you?"
- Seek only enough information to formulate a suspicion. Do not interrogate.
- Immediately report *all* suspicions of child abuse to the proper authorities. Do not examine the child unless there is a specific complaint of injury or pain.

- Insist on counseling for child and parent.
- Work with police and community agencies.
- Insist that staff report suspicions to the proper authorities.
- Document objectively according to your district and state regulations so there is no room for multiple interpretations.
- Do *not* allow a child to go home to an unsafe environment. Do *not* transport a child in your car. Consult local law enforcement agency for assistance.
- Do *not* call *the parents* unless directed to do so by the protective agency.
- If the investigator from the child protective services agency feels that an investigation is not warranted and you strongly disagree, speak with another investigator or supervisor. Keep asking for an investigation until someone listens.
- Keep notes on the referral in a confidential file. It may be necessary to retrieve this information years later.

References

Centers for Disease Control and Prevention. (2013). *Child abuse and neglect prevention.* Retrieved from https://www.cdc.gov/violenceprevention/childabuseandneglect/index.html

Child Welfare Information Gateway. (2007). *Definitions of child abuse and neglect in Federal Law.* Retrieved from https://www.childwelfare.gov/topics/can/defining/federal/

Child Welfare Information Gateway. (2013). *What is child abuse and neglect? Recognizing the signs and symptoms.* Retrieved from https://www.childwelfare.gov/pubs/factsheets/whatiscan/

Child Welfare Information Gateway. (2017). *About CAPTA: A legislative history.* Washington, DC: U.S. Department of Health and Human Services, Children's Bureau.

National Children's Advocacy Center. (2010). *Physical and behavioral indicators of abuse.* Retrieved from http://www.nationalcac.org

V

Problems Unique to the School Nurse Setting

20

School Violence and Disaster Planning

Every nurse knows what an emergency is. Nurses have been educated and are ready to recognize a serious threat, deal with the acute phase, help in the recovery process, and then work to prevent future similar incidents by reflecting on the why and how of the emergency.

In school nursing practice, nurses have emergency plans for certain students. We know exactly what must be done for a child who is anaphylactic, diabetic, or has a seizure disorder. There are clear protocols for children with special needs as well as for anticipated schoolwide emergencies such as fires and structural issues.

Nurses and many other school personnel are certified in cardiopulmonary resuscitation and automatic external defibrillator use. These skills are seldom, if ever, needed, but we are prepared in case they are.

Most school emergency situations can be planned for, responded to, and recovered from, all within the school community. A large disaster or mass casualty cannot be managed in the same way, as the needs far exceed the limited resources of the school and district.

In this chapter, you will learn:

1. The definition of a safe school
2. The types of disasters and actions that need to be taken.

3. The stages of disaster planning and preparing a GoKit
4. Causes of violence in today's schools

A SAFE SCHOOL

In the hierarchy of needs, safety comes well before learning. We know that children can and will learn only if they feel protected. Today's schools are an integral part of the community and must be a refuge for students.

Every school district is required to have a well-written and frequently rehearsed plan that covers all the different types of mass emergencies and traumatic events. This plan should specify the courses of action for students and staff so all can effectively respond to the crisis. Every response must be tailored to the type of incident so valuable time is not lost.

Each local board of education is given the task of establishing policies and procedures to ensure that a sense of peace and stability remains constant in schools so that learning can take place.

Fast Facts

One of the first tasks you should explore when you begin work in a school district is to carefully check the safety plans for fire and mass disasters.

Clinical Snapshot

On the morning of September 11, 2001, anxious calls flooded every school in the nation. Parents sought reassurance that their children were within the safety of the school walls. Terribly shaken, many parents left their homes or workplaces to go to their children's schools so that they could see and touch their children and know they were unharmed.

The police, firefighters, and social services organizations mobilized. Hospitals near Ground Zero in New York City immediately prepared to discharge as many patients as possible to make room for anticipated casualties. Medical care facilities within the general area braced themselves for an onslaught of patients. Much of the world responded to the crisis in some manner, offering to provide any needed assistance.

Fortunately, disasters such as this are rare. However, just as we prepare for fires with fire drills and for classroom emergencies with student emergency care plans, we must also be prepared for a major catastrophe.

There are many components to a safe school, and a multidisciplinary team approach is essential. Schools must partner with police, fire workers, and rescue workers. The school nurse must participate in all such approaches and assume a prominent role.

Healthy People 2020 Objectives:
Preparedness, 2:
Reduce the time necessary to activate designated personnel to report for immediate duty with no advance notice from 66 minutes in 2009 to 59 minutes.

TYPES OF DISASTERS

Violence

A violent disaster involves an act of shooting, bomb planting, or suicide. Schools must recognize that bullying, depression, and self-destructive behavior are increasing. Every threat must be taken seriously and the person posing a threat referred immediately.

Schools must have a lockdown plan for the violent intruder. Bomb threats require immediate evacuation to designated safe areas. Every bomb threat should be dealt with by immediate evacuation of all students and staff.

Terrorism and Bioterrorism

In the wake of 9/11, acts of terrorism are the foremost fear of many Americans today. One type of terrorism is bioterrorism, which is the release of small amounts of toxic biological substances that can cause tremendous harm. Table 20.1 summarizes the classification of biological agents of concern.

Table 20.1

Classification of Biological Agents

Risk Category	Characteristics of Agents
Category A agents (highest priority risk)	
Botulinum toxin (*Clostridium botulinum*)	■ Easily disseminated or transmitted from person to person
Plague (*Yersinia pestis*)	■ High morbidity and mortality rates
Smallpox (*Variola major*)	■ Major health impact

(continued)

Table 20.1

Classification of Biological Agents (*continued*)

Risk Category	Characteristics of Agents
Category A agents (highest priority risk) (*continued*)	
Tularemia (*Francisella tularensis*)	■ Potential for public panic and social disruption
Viral hemorrhagic fevers (including Ebola, Marburg, Lassa, and Machupo)	■ Require special action for public health preparedness
Category B agents (second-highest priority risk)	
Brucellosis	■ Moderately easy to disseminate
Epsilon toxin of *Clostridium perfringens*	■ Results in moderate morbidity rates and low mortality rates
Food safety threats (*Salmonella, Escherichia coli, Shigella*); melioidosis, psittacosis (*Chlamydia psittaci*); Q fever (*Coxiella burnetii*); ricin toxin (from castor beans)	■ Require specific enhancements of CDC's diagnostic capacity and enhanced disease surveillance
Staphylococcal enterotoxin B; typhus fever (*Rickettsia prowazekii*); viral encephalitis (from alphaviruses such as VEE, EEE, WEE)	
Category C agents (third-highest priority risk)	
Emerging infectious diseases such as Nipah virus and hantavirus	■ Availability ■ Ease of production and dissemination ■ Potential for high morbidity and mortality rates and major health impact

CDC, Centers for Disease Control and Prevention; EEE, Eastern equine encephalomyelitis; VEE, Venezuelan equine encephalomyelitis; WEE, Western equine encephalomyelitis.

Source: Centers for Disease Control and Prevention. Bioterrorism agents/diseases. (2018). Retrieved from https://emergency.cdc.gov/agent/agentlist-category.asp.

Natural and Environmental Disasters

Hurricanes, floods, earthquakes, and tornados can all be natural disasters impacting schools. Although no one is to blame for such disasters, their effects are frightening and devastating, as are the effects of environmental disasters. Examples of environmental disasters include toxic exposures or spills and structural failure of a school building.

In the event of a natural disaster, students should be directed to a safe part of the building and advised to duck and cover their heads. All hazardous material releases should entail an immediate, forced evacuation.

Fire or Explosion

School fires are not uncommon, and today we have mandatory evacuation drills.

Illness

Any illness that strikes a significant percentage of the population can cause a crisis. Large numbers of people with pandemic flu or similar difficult-to-control illnesses are considered to be disasters in a community.

If a child is diagnosed by a physician with a disease that we have an immunization for, this must be reported to the local and/or state health departments.

Also catastrophic is the sudden death of a student or staff member. Suicides are especially tragic and may involve copy-cat behaviors. Be alert for the individuals who have expressed suicidal thoughts, friends and colleagues close to the person who has died.

Carefully monitor reports of highly contagious diseases. Immediately exclude children exhibiting symptoms of contagious diseases. Keep the administration, the school medical officer, and parents informed. Always advise parents to discuss concerns with their private physicians.

CAUSES OF VIOLENT BEHAVIOR IN TODAY'S SCHOOLS

Violence of any type is a multifaceted problem, which makes identifying a specific cause almost impossible. However, we can speculate on a number of possibilities that have caused this to be a major threat to our children.

Recent years have seen a dramatic increase in the number of deaths on school grounds. Most agree that school violence comes from a layering of different risk factors. Possible causes include:

- Access to guns
- Unstable family life
- Poverty

- Mental illness
- Media violence
- Gang influence
- Cyber abuse

Fast Facts

Violence is defined as the intentional use of physical force or power against another person, group, or community with the behavior likely to cause physical or psychological harm (Centers for Disease Control and Prevention [CDC], 2014). A violent act always has a victim, who can be another student, a teacher, or a staff member. A student might be a victim, a perpetrator, or both.

The sad truth is that as long as violence occurs in our society, it will also occur in our schools. Schools simply mirror what is going on in the community or larger world.

Clinical Snapshot

Joseph is a student with severe behavioral issues. He is one of a number of 10th graders who belong to a gang allegedly responsible for numerous acts of violence in the community. School nurse Sharon is aware that he has served time in a juvenile detention center and is now returning to school on probation. Sharon must be part of the team planning his re-entrance back to the school community. Careful monitoring is essential here.

WHAT CAN BE DONE?

Student movements such as Enough Is Enough (#Never Again) have raised the consciousness of the nation. Following a mass shooting of 16 students and one teacher in Coral Springs, Florida, in 2018, many students throughout the country demonstrated in support of better gun control.

Many also believe that more funds must be made available to research the correlation between gun violence and gun availability as a cause of death in our nation.

Others believe differently. In 1996, Congress passed the Dickey Amendment mandating that no CDC funds could be spent on research that may be used to advocate or promote gun control.

In 2005, Congress passed the Protection of Lawful Commerce in Arms Act shielding gun manufacturers and sellers from civil claim brought by victims of gun violence.

DISASTER PLANNING

Factors to Consider

- The total number of people involved: students, staff, and anticipated visitors
- The number of students and staff members with special needs; note those who are wheelchair bound
- The type of disaster
- Evacuation plans
- Assembly points
- Means of communication

STAFF TRAINING

Crisis Team Members

Each local board of education must establish policies and procedures to deal with crises. The chief school administrator must put together a crisis team.

Fast Facts

A crisis team must:

- Serve as an advisory board to the chief school administrator
- Inform school personnel of information as it develops
- Deliver services as needed

Clinical Snapshot

School nurse Sharon notes that the crisis team is planning to meet later in the afternoon. When she approaches her principal about the time and location, she is told that it is not necessary for her to attend and that there is no one to cover her office. Sharon explains the importance of her presence and suggests they try to get a substitute nurse for a couple of hours or direct the staff to send only emergencies and inform the secretary where she could be reached. Sharon feels strongly that since she is part of the solution, she should be included in the planning.

School Members

- Chief school administrator
- School psychologist

- All principals in the district
- School nurse
- Director of buildings and grounds
- Bus driver
- Guidance counselor
- Special education teacher
- School secretary
- Custodian
- Parents' organization representative
- Social worker
- Regular education teacher

Community Members

- Police department
- Fire department
- Community mental health personnel
- Emergency services personnel
- Local public officials
- Parents
- Representatives of local medical facilities

Fast Facts

Keep all disaster information and equipment in a location that is easy to access. Make sure your administrator is aware of the location, and include the location in your substitute nurse's folder.

Clinical Snapshot

Sharon has an office the size of a large closet. Her *GoKit* and other crisis necessities simply do not fit in an accessible location. It is crucial that space be allocated for these items. Perhaps a shelf can be added, or a space in a nearby classroom can be designated for these essential emergency tools.

PLANNING STAGES AND SCHOOL NURSES' ROLE

There are four stages in becoming prepared for and responding to the variety of school disasters that may take place within your school environment:

1. Identify potential disasters (for your school environment)
2. Be prepared (for possible disaster types)

3. Respond (appropriately to the disaster)
4. Recover (provide recovery support, as needed)

   A detailed description of these stages follows.

Identify Potential Disasters

This is primary prevention when it is most important. There is little anyone can do to avert terrorism, natural disasters, or even many environmental issues. However, violence can and should be addressed more effectively in the schools.

Role of School Nurses in Identifying Potential Disasters

- Help create a school climate that fosters an atmosphere of respect between adults and students.
- Consider offering schoolwide safety and character-education programs.
- Insist on a no-bullying policy, and see that it is enforced.
- Watch the loners. Every student should fit in with someone.
- Be alert for threats.
- Find students who will inform you of classmates who make threats and are willing to break the students' code of silence.
- Insist on written physician clearance for any student returning to school after a period of depression or suicide attempt, stating that the student is not a danger to self or others.

Be Prepared

In preparation for a disaster, it is essential that consideration be given to general disaster principles and specific plans for individual schools. Each school has a different location, types and ages of students, and individual needs that will influence emergency planning.

The School Emergency Plan

The school emergency plan should be reviewed annually and updated as needed. Drills should be practiced at least yearly, meet the unique needs of the individual school, and delegate specific activities for each member of the crisis team. In addition, the school emergency plan should include the following:

- An outline of a predetermined response plan
- Provisions for trained people with knowledge and skills to act as emergency responders
- Provisions to minimize the risk of serious injury, death, or property damage

- Provisions for first aid and counseling for staff, students, parents, and community members during and after the crisis
- Provisions for accurate, up-to-date information to be given to parents, the community, and the media
- Guidelines for how to evaluate the response and revise the plan
- A goal to return the school to its normal level of function as soon as possible
- Development of a post-emergency plan for the aftermath of any disaster

Types of School Disaster Drills

- *Evacuation*: The students must exit the building in a quick, orderly fashion, as for a threat of a fire.
- *Lockdown*: A lockdown is necessary when a perpetrator is believed to be present in the building or on the school grounds. Students are directed to stand clear of doors and windows, and rooms are locked.
- *Drop and cover*: Students are directed to take shelter under desks or against walls, with their bodies covered as much as possible. This is recommended during a natural disaster such as a hurricane or tornado.

Role of School Nurses in Preparing for a Disaster

- Ask to review the school emergency plan.
- Be part of the crisis management team.
- Assemble a school nurse's GoKit (Table 20.2).

Table 20.2

School Nurse's GoKit Components

Documents	
Crisis management plan	School blueprints
Emergency cards	Individualized and emergency plans
Teacher and student class lists	Absentee list for the day
Alert list	Standing orders
Medication list for students and staff	Emergency evacuation plans
Class pictures or yearbook	Important phone numbers
Supplies	
Emergency medications	Daily medications
Students' personal medications	Spill kit
Gloves, gowns	Bandages, splints, ice packs

(continued)

Table 20.2

School Nurse's GoKit Components (*continued*)

Supplies	
Biohazard bags and masks	Flashlight
Communication devices	Blood pressure machine, stethoscope
Master keys for building	Hand sanitizer
Pens, paper, markers	Name tags, triage tags

Respond

Once the traumatic event has occurred, intervention takes place. Ideally, plans are in place, procedures have been rehearsed, and the team is ready and available to protect the students.

Role of School Nurses in Responding to a Disaster

- Organize the first-aid treatment for the injured.
- Triage.
- Counsel students as needed while remaining calm.
- Make sure that those with special needs are tended to.
- Keep your GoKit with you.

Recovery

After the crisis situation has passed, the school community enters the recovery phase. This is a critical time for all, and the school nurse's calm effectiveness will be vital to the community.

Role of School Nurses in Recovering From a Disaster

- Provide opportunities for people to come together. This will allow them to grasp the situation better.
- Provide reassurance that the crisis has passed and that students are safe.
- Openly share what information you have.
- Support parents and teachers so they can support students as they recover from the trauma.

Fast Facts

Disasters do happen. When or if a disaster occurs in your school, you will be a key player. Make sure you prepare in every possible way.

(*continued*)

(continued)

Clinical Snapshot

Sharon seldom is absent. When her mom became ill, she needed to take several days off to care for her. Fortunately, she had oriented her substitute nurse, office secretary, and building principal well concerning her crisis plans. She was able to take off to handle her personal crisis, knowing that a plan was in place in the event of a schoolwide emergency.

Reference

Centers for Disease Control and Prevention. (2014). *Elder abuse: Definitions.* Retrieved from www.cdc.gov/violenceprevention/elderabuse/definitions.html

21

Environmental Issues

All children have the right to attend a school that is environmentally healthy and completely safe. No parent, teacher, or administrator would disagree with this statement.

Health and safety are intertwined; one cannot exist without the other. Learning cannot and will not *take place unless these basic needs are met.*

Increasingly educators are focusing on the impact of the environment on students' health and their ability to learn. Water, air quality, and environmental hazards affect everyone, including a school's many occupants. The knowledge base about environmental issues continues to grow and become ever more complex.

School is the child's and staff's second home. Today's school day begins earlier for many and goes into the evening with after care and special events. Many occupants could easily be exposed to harmful toxins found in molds, asbestos, drinking water, cleaning products, food, or pesticides.

In this chapter, you will learn:

1. Concerns about toxins and the state of school buildings today
2. The four areas of concern in the school environment and specific toxins that may pose threats to the school environment
3. The reasons why children are more susceptible than adults to environmental toxins
4. Preventive strategies to deal with environmental toxins

ENVIRONMENTAL TOXINS

Environmental toxins have been blamed for triggering the onset of acute and chronic illnesses. Children and teachers who are ill are frequently absent, and when they are in school, they are not able to work at their full potential—learning is compromised and delayed.

The environment continues to evolve, and we all adapt to changing circumstances. It is the job of school personnel to educate children despite any obstacles. A healthful school environment is one of the eight components of a coordinated school health program. In this area, as in many others, school nurses can play a significant role in the prevention, detection, and early correction of environmental health issues.

Healthy People 2020 Objectives:
Environmental Health, 16.1:
Increase the proportion of the nation's elementary, middle, and high schools that have an indoor air quality management program to promote a healthy and safe physical school environment from 51.4% in 2006 to 56.5%.

TODAY'S SCHOOL BUILDINGS

In recent years, there has been increasing concern about the conditions of school buildings. Most of these structures were built in the early 1900s with an anticipated life span of 50 to 100 years. These buildings have withstood decades of abuse, neglect, and conditions of terrible overcrowding. They have served generations of children well, but today many are in need of repair or replacement.

The majority of other school facilities were built in the 1960s or 1970s and had an anticipated life span of only about 30 years. They have also served students well but need to be repaired or to be razed and rebuilt.

Many of both types of buildings are nearing their maximum life expectancy simultaneously at a time when funding is scarce or nonexistent. The cost of building new facilities, especially with all of the new federal and state requirements, is astronomical, and repairing these outdated facilities is simply not feasible.

Unfortunately, in many cases, school buildings have not been well maintained. Tax money designated for school expenses has often gone to rising fuel and electricity costs, contracted teachers' salaries, escalating insurance costs, or newly mandated programs. School building maintenance has simply not been a priority.

When absolutely necessary, new school facilities are constructed. However, these present their own issues. The soil must be free of contaminants, the location must be away from noise, and numerous building codes must be carefully adhered to.

Consequently, school systems today are dealing with deteriorating buildings that present opportunities for all kinds of health issues. As these issues are resolved, new ones continue to surface.

Fast Facts

Outside of home, children spend more time in school than in any other place. Many children today are enrolled in before-school care programs and often stay well beyond the regular school day for after-school care, sports, or social events. The average student spends over 14,000 total hours in school from kindergarten through grade 12.

Clinical Snapshot

Mrs. L. is concerned about her 6-year-old daughter, Lisa. Because of both parents' work schedules, Lisa participates in the before- and after-school programs, spending almost 12 hours every day in the school building. Lisa has numerous allergies to airborne toxins and various foods. Mrs. L. would like assurance from you that the prolonged school presence will not harm her child and that medical attention will be available if necessary. School nurse Ellen informs Mrs. L. that in your school, the before- and after-care program is run independently and that you are not in the building the entire time. When present, you will do all you can to protect Lisa, as you do the other children. Ellen suggests that Mrs. L speak to the before- and after-school providers and, if she is not comfortable, that she consider other childcare options.

THE SCHOOL ENVIRONMENT

At a minimum, schools should be expected to have the following:

- Clean air, free from dust and mold
- Adequate climate control and ventilation
- No mold present
- Freedom from violence
- Healthful food and clean drinking water
- No harmful bacteria or chemical dust

- Intact roofs and ceilings
- Safe stairwells and, if present, working elevators
- Well-maintained playground equipment on nontoxic soil
- Intact sidewalks, walls, and foundations
- Private, clean, working sinks, toilets, and adequate soap and paper towels

There are a number of areas in our schools where the school nurse needs to concern himself or herself about environmental safety. These include:

1. The building's physical structure: Playground, shop, lunchroom, classrooms, fields, heating and cooling systems, sidewalks
2. The people who occupy the building: Students, staff, visitors
3. Equipment: Room dividers, bleachers, cleaning supplies, gym equipment
4. Activities: Field trips, busing, eating, gym activities

SPECIFIC TOXINS

There are a wide variety of potentially threatening toxins in schools and on school property. The following toxins, if present in the school environment, can cause skin eruptions, respiratory distress, organ damage, central nervous system symptoms, cancer, mesothelioma, allergic reaction, headaches, or a variety of other symptoms depending on the source. Today our concerns are focused on the following toxins.

Asbestos

Asbestos is any of several minerals that readily separate into long, flexible fibers and have been implicated as causes of certain types of cancers.

Schools that were built before 1980 most likely will contain some form of asbestos. If the asbestos materials are in good condition, the Environmental Protection Agency insists that they pose insignificant risk and recommends that the asbestos not be removed. If removal is necessary, there is a proper procedure to be followed. Asbestos can be present in ceiling tiles, vinyl flooring, or used for pipe wrappings. Premature death and mesothelioma are linked to asbestos exposures.

Mold

Mold is a fungal, wooly growth that forms on damp or decaying organic matter. Without proper ventilation, mold can develop in less than 72 hours. During the summer months, classrooms are not inspected daily. Damp ceiling tiles, carpeting, or fabrics can become mold substrates. The mold reproduces quickly by creating spores that are airborne and targets lungs and skin, causing irritation. Students might also complain of headache, rash, fatigue, nausea, and eye, skin, and respiratory irritation. Frequent inspections and proper ventilation will help control mold spread.

Lead

Lead can enter drinking water when pipes that contain lead begin to corrode. Many of our older schools were built when pipes were not lead free. Today the Centers for Disease Control and Prevention (CDC) recommends that public health actions be initiated when the level of lead in a child's blood is 5 mcg/dL or more. Many pediatricians include lead level testing as part of a routine physical exam. Even low levels can lead to behavior and learning problems, lower IQ, slow growth, and anemia.

Environmentally Triggered Illnesses

These are illnesses that are reactions to common elements in a person's environment: food, chemicals, water, and tiny physical particles. Symptoms can involve multiple organs of the body, resulting in a poor state of health.

Sick-Building Syndrome

This term describes a situation in which a building occupant experiences acute symptoms linked to the time spent in the building but no specific illness can be identified. Headaches and eye, ear, nose, and throat irritations are common. Poor ventilation or chemical contaminants are usually the cause. Symptoms subside once the person leaves the building.

CAUSES OF SUSCEPTIBILITY IN CHILDREN

Schools have become community centers. They house preschool and special needs programs, offer extended school days, and are used throughout the year. It is important now more than ever that their environments be healthy.

Fast Facts

If you are suspicious that the school environment might be causing or exacerbating illness in your students and staff, begin to note the location, time, and symptoms displayed. Compare your notes for different parts of the building.

Clinical Snapshot

Carlos is a fifth-grade student known to have multiple airborne allergies. He frequently sees Ellen during the day with watery eyes and a sore throat. His mom reports that he does not have symptoms at home. Ellen has had no other complaints from students or parents.

Complaints of this nature should be reported to the school physician and administration and followed up with the local board of health.

Every growing child reacts differently when exposed to toxins, and children, in general, have a much lower tolerance than adults do. Sometimes, symptoms of illness can go undetected for years. Some reasons why children are more susceptible than adults are described in the following sections.

Medical Fragility

The health of children with special needs may be compromised by additional factors, such as medication use and immobility issues.

Body Size and Weight

Because children are smaller in height and weight than adults, toxins become more concentrated in their bodies. Since their body systems are developing, they are more susceptible to toxins, and extra care must be taken to provide a safe and protective school environment.

Metabolism

Children metabolize food and toxins quickly, and their bodies respond rapidly.

Nutritional Status

Often, children do not eat properly. They may come to school without an adequate breakfast and have little energy in reserve. Swift and competent assessment of potential toxin exposure and appropriate follow-up care is imperative to protect children from avoidable adverse effects on their health.

Underdeveloped Immune System

Children's immune systems develop as the children do. Very young children have less, if any, immunity to foreign toxins.

Immature Brain and Central Nervous System

The nervous systems of children continue to develop as they age. Their brains are highly susceptible to assaults by foreign substances that enter their bodies.

PREVENTION STRATEGIES

As with every other aspect of health, prevention is the key. This is best accomplished through an organized preventive safety and health program. Such a program might include the following measures:

- Implementing a comprehensive school health education program in which preventive health measures (e.g., handwashing, control of communicable diseases) are taught in an organized, sequential manner
- Offering annual staff education covering the recognition of anaphylaxis or any allergic responses as well as information about blood-borne pathogens
- Insisting on the routine inspection of the building and playground equipment for structural safety
- Developing guidelines for appropriate handling of animals in the classroom
- Recommending that construction work, major cleaning, painting, and lawn services be done when the building is not occupied by students
- Setting up a proper reporting system for handling environmental concerns
- Checking to see that classrooms are clean, are at a comfortable temperature, and are well ventilated
- Insisting on a no-smoking policy in the school and on the grounds

- Not permitting buses or cars to idle close to the school, where exhaust fumes can be inhaled
- Keeping careful documentation so that patterns of illnesses can be detected

ESTABLISHMENT OF LAWS AND AGENCIES DESIGNED TO PROTECT THE ENVIRONMENT

Concerns about a safe and healthy school environment have prompted the development of laws and agencies specifically designed to protect children (Table 21.1).

ROLE OF SCHOOL NURSES IN ENVIRONMENTAL ISSUES

- Be alert for groups of students exhibiting vague constitutional symptoms.
- Monitor, report, and intervene to correct any hazard.
- Develop individualized healthcare, emergency care, or 504 plans to address each child's specific sensitivities.
- Have an exposure control plan in place.
- Be prepared to handle and triage a massive environmental crisis.
- Know the laws governing environmental issues in your state and district.

Table 21.1

Timeline of Major Legislation and Agency Formation Established to Protect the Environment

1970	Environmental Protection Agency: Agency of the federal government charged with protecting the health and environment for all people
1970	Occupational Safety and Health Act: Protects employees from a work environment containing health hazards
1986	The Asbestos Hazard Emergency Response Act: Requires public and private schools to inspect school buildings for asbestos and to remove the asbestos appropriately
1991	Occupational Safety and Health Act: Established rules to protect employees from potential exposure to blood and other body fluids
1994	Pro-Children Act: Prohibits indoor smoking in places used to provide educational services to children younger than 18 years

- Participate in committees to assess plans and implement environmental safety programs.
- Support legislation to improve environmental health.
- Offer in-service education to all staff.
- Communicate effectively with students, staff, and the administration regarding clusters of physical ailments.
- Keep detailed notes on all reports of environmental issues.
- Support school funding for construction and renovation projects.
- Be fully prepared to act in the event of an environmental emergency.

Fast Facts

Because of the close relationship with staff, students, parents, and members of the community, the school nurse can have a key role in prevention and early detection of harmful toxins in the school environment.

Clinical Snapshot

Ellen notes that four students and two teachers were recently diagnosed with pneumonia. All have their homerooms located in a separate wing of the building with its own forced-air heating system. Ellen reports the statistics to the building administrator, school physician, and local health department. Air quality testing may be in order.

22

Technology in the School Health Office

If today's school nurses were granted three wishes relevant to their jobs, they would probably be (a) less paperwork, (b) more time to spend with students, and (c) even less paperwork and even more time to spend with students. Thus far, the school nurse genie has not appeared for any of us, so we must work with what is actually available.

Technology can provide school nurses with assistance in streamlining health office paperwork. The catch is that the transition from paperwork to electronic documents will initially involve time and effort.

In this chapter, you will learn:

1. Rationale and basic uses for computers in the school health office
2. Advantages and disadvantages of a paperless health office
3. Technological equipment currently in use
4. Technical terminology
5. Steps for incorporating computers in the health office

RATIONALE

It might be helpful to keep in mind that school nursing is a specialty of the nursing profession. By definition, this means that, as professionals, school nurses continue to learn. If any of us were to see a child with an illness we had never heard of, without hesitation, we would gather information, assess the data, make a plan about how to help the patient, implement the plan, and periodically evaluate the patient and the plan for effectiveness. School nurses follow the nursing process to do their jobs effectively so that patients have good outcomes.

If school nurses lack knowledge about anything relevant to their professional performance, they must study and learn to be proficient. Computer skills are no different.

School nurses who began their careers without the use of computers might struggle and resist this new challenge. Those who were immediately comfortable with technology must contend with those who do not have the same level of expertise. If you are part of the first group, you must change. If you are part of the latter group, consider taking a leadership role to help your colleagues.

You have probably already developed a network of reliable resources to support you in your practice. You know whom to call for answers to certain questions. You have modeled your nursing and teaching style after those whom you admire and respect. Now you may need a technical coach to guide you. By embracing this new challenge, you will find freedom from many tedious tasks and the opportunity to spend more of your valuable time educating and helping students.

Healthy People 2020 Objectives:
Health Communication and Health
Information Technology, 6.1:
Increase the proportion of persons with access to
the Internet from 68.5% in 2007 to 75.4%.

USES OF COMPUTER TECHNOLOGY IN SCHOOL HEALTH OFFICES

There are three primary uses for computers in the health office:

1. Keeping logs (medication and daily)
2. Writing reports (monthly and annual)
3. Maintaining records (cumulative and immunization)

ADVANTAGES AND DISADVANTAGES OF A PAPERLESS HEALTH OFFICE

Most hospitals do some or all documentation electronically, and efficiently run businesses rely on technology to deliver comprehensive services to clients. Schools and their health offices are no different. Some of the advantages and disadvantages of a computerized and paperless health office are described in the following sections.

Advantages

- Information is stored, added, and easily retrieved as needed.
- Screening rosters can be printed, and documents can be scanned.
- Access is limited, so privacy can be maintained.
- Tabulation of information for reports and referrals is easy.
- Memos and letters to parents can be personalized for distribution.
- Transfer of information is easier.
- Research can be done via the Internet to reduce the number of costly reference books.
- School nurses can be quickly connected with other school nurses across the country and throughout the world.
- New school nurses can be oriented via specific teaching modules.
- Information can be accessed immediately, from any site at any time.

Disadvantages

- It can be difficult to find the exact software package to meet each nurse's needs.
- New, advanced computers are constantly being developed, and some cannot be updated.
- Training is needed, and help must be available to troubleshoot problems.
- Confidentiality remains a concern. School nurses and office personnel have an ethical responsibility to protect the integrity of electronic student health records from both accidental and malicious tampering. Passwords are needed.
- All data must be backed up.

Fast Facts

You are already a savvy user of many technological devices. Now it is time to expand this knowledge to help you even more in the health office.

Clinical Snapshot

Virginia was a school nurse in a small district where she did not even have a computer. She now works in a large urban district with other nurses who have varying degrees of technical ability.

Use a team approach when dealing with technology issues. Seek in-service programs for all the nurses in your county or district, and try to agree on the best program for all. This will provide continuity for substitute nurses and transient students and as children move through the system.

ELECTRONIC EQUIPMENT CURRENTLY IN USE

Most school nurses are already technically adept to some degree. Many use the equipment described in the following sections to receive and transmit student health information.

Cell Phones and Cordless Phones

It is hard to imagine life before cell phones and cordless phones. Many school districts provide nurses with cell phones to carry with them so that they are accessible throughout the day.

Personal Digital Assistant

This is a small battery-powered computer. Used with a stylus, similar to a small pencil, it can exchange data with another computer. Nurses like personal digital assistants because they can easily be carried in their pockets.

Voice Mail

Voice mail allows people to leave messages for school nurses regarding student absences, illnesses, parental conferences, and so on. Nurses also leave voice mail messages alerting parents to concerns about their children during the school day.

Fax Machines

Fax machines and scanners are now used to transmit health information. They are most helpful in obtaining doctors' orders, parental consents, immunization dates, health records, and medication data. A health-related fax must include a cover page stating that the information being transmitted is confidential and has limited use by authorized personnel. The fax machine should be in a secure area accessible only to the school nurse and authorized staff. The nurse must be aware of any state or district policy that requires original, signed documents for doctors' orders.

Fast Facts

Some guidelines to keep in mind for the use of fax machines include the following:

- Fax only when time demands it.
- Send and receive only information that is necessary.

(continued)

(continued)

- Keep communications short.
- Remember to obtain authorization.

Clinical Snapshot

There is only one fax machine in the school building's main office. All have access to it. When sending or receiving confidential medical information, Virginia makes sure it is marked as such and insists that no one sort these incoming faxes.

If possible, a separate fax should be provided for your exclusive use.

Answering Machines

An answering machine delivers a prerecorded message to callers and saves their messages until the school nurse listens to and deletes them. This allows the nurse to take calls when there are no other priorities.

Email

It is important to have parental permission before using email regarding any student. Parents must be informed that this information may be added to their child's permanent health record. There should be a confidentiality statement on all messages regarding students. For all other internal school communication, email is an efficient, time-saving method of communication.

COMPUTER COMPONENTS

Computers are composed of external and internal parts. These include:

- Screen or monitor to visualize the information
- Tower containing the "brains" of the computer
- Keyboard
- Mouse—the physical object that moves and controls a pointer or display on the screen
- *Optional components:*
- Printer to transfer screen information onto paper or hard copy
  - Removable media devices to store information
  - Compact disc
  - Flash drive

TECHNICAL TERMINOLOGY

The following information was adapted from Saugus (1998) and defines some technological terms that are commonly used.

- Boot-up: To start the computer
- Crash: Unintentional shutting down of the computer
- Bug: A mistake in design of software
- Firewall: Part of the computer that restricts data from flowing through
- Search engine: A service that allows Internet users to search for content via the World Wide Web
- Software: Data or program
- Spam: Unsolicited email messages
- Virus: A program that can harm the computer

THE INTERNET

The Internet is the worldwide network of linked computers that provides users with access to information on the World Wide Web as well as email and file transfer services. Today's school nurse can send information and messages electronically to a parent a few blocks away sitting at his or her desk or across the world into cyberspace, the theoretical boundary of the Internet.

TELEHEALTH

Telehealth assists the school nurse in two ways. It permits the school nurse to communicate with a healthcare provider to discuss a child's needs and attend lectures or educational programs offered where she cannot physically be present. It is especially useful in rural areas and is popular as a long-distance teaching tool.

STEPS TO CONVERT TO A COMPUTERIZED HEALTH OFFICE

The easiest, most effective method of transitioning to a computerized, paperless health office is to apply the five steps of the nursing process: data collection, assessment, planning and goal setting, implementation, and evaluation.

Data Collection

As a school nurse, one of your goals is to gain insight into your strengths and the needs of your colleagues. Start by organizing a meeting in which you all brainstorm your concerns about paperwork. Get a sense of other nurses' attitudes and abilities related to computer use.

Assessment

Review and analyze the data you have collected. Consider finances and resources that will be available to you. Discuss your concerns with any available experts: staff members of technology departments in your school district, administrators, and nurses in other districts who have already initiated programs.

Planning and Goal Setting

Set reasonable goals. Perhaps you plan to initiate a computerized program in just one school in the district. You may need to visit another health office to see how the system works. Computer and software companies sometimes send representatives to lead in-service educational programs. Check to see if you are eligible for such a program. Formulate short- and long-term plans of action.

Implementation

Carry out the initial short-term plan of action under whatever terms you have agreed upon. Try one new task at a time, and do not be afraid to make a mistake. You might begin by simply printing class rosters for screening purposes or generating memos.

Evaluation

Revisit your goals to see if the actual outcome matches the intended one. If your goal was to obtain a computer for every health office and only half the offices have them, find out why. Can the situation be remedied? Perhaps the goal was to have all nurses attend a training workshop, but some were not able to. Explore options for training those nurses. Reconsider the goals you made, and formulate new ones to move forward.

ROLE OF SCHOOL NURSES IN TECHNOLOGY

- Accept the new challenges of technology.
- Be willing to attend workshops or take courses to learn how to use equipment.
- Seek and accept technology assistance whenever possible.
- Protect the privacy of computerized health information as you would any medical documents.

Fast Facts

Technology is new, different, and difficult for those who were not raised in the computer generation. It is *not* impossible to learn. Be patient with yourself. You have done harder things.

Clinical Snapshot

Virginia is a warm, caring, highly competent school nurse. She struggles with use of the computer in the health office and, intending to retire in a few years, is reluctant to learn. As a professional person who is relied upon to perform at a certain level, she must make every effort to reach out for technical knowledge and support so she can fulfill her professional obligations.

Reference

Saugus.net. (1998). *Glossary of Computer Terms*. Retrieved from https://www.saugus.net/Computer/Terms/

23

Top 10 Troublesome Topics for the School Nurse

The greatest challenge school nurses face today may lie not with the ever-changing knowledge base or how we deliver healthcare, but with the day-to-day situations unique to our profession. Some issues hang over school nurses, draining and depleting us of needed energy for the more important tasks involved in direct student care.

In this chapter, 10 of these frustrating issues are addressed. Certainly, there are no simple solutions for all of these problems. However, it is appropriate to share some suggestions in hopes that they will prove useful and support school nurses in recognizing that they are not alone.

TOPIC 1: LACK OF SCHOOL NURSE SUBSTITUTES

Fast Facts

If there is one common complaint all school nurses share, it is the lack of competent substitutes to care for students in our absence. We can assume that coverage has always been a concern, but since the passage of legislation requiring students with special needs to be placed in *the least restrictive environment*, many good, caring

(continued)

(*continued*)

nurses, recognizing that greater skills would be required in the school setting, have become fearful of working independently in a school. This situation has become a crisis for many nurses and school districts.

Clinical Snapshot

School nurses shared the following experiences, describing situations in which they could not arrange for coverage:

- *Hannah came to work with a temperature of 102°F to check on a child with diabetes and give out medications.*
- Stephanie had to miss her son's graduation.
- *Jenna spent 15 minutes on the phone in the emergency department, trying to find a sub while her father was experiencing chest pain.*
- *A student in Kim's school had a seizure while she was working at another school she had been sent to cover.*
- *Camila waited months for approval to attend a workshop, paid for it herself, and arranged for a sub. While standing on line at the conference registration desk, she received a call from the principal, directing her to return to school immediately. The sub had cancelled.*

Suggested School Nurse Actions

A. Lobby to raise the pay for school nurse substitutes:
   - Coordinate with other districts to ensure that all substitute nurses receive pay equivalent to a per diem rate from a local agency.
   - Insist on a paid orientation for all new school nurse substitutes.

B. Recruit:
   - If some of the mothers of children in your school are registered professional nurses and you know and trust them, ask them to consider substituting for you.
   - Call the director of nursing programs at your local university or college with bachelor's and master's programs for registered nurses, and ask if any students might be interested in working as substitutes.
   - Borrow a substitute from another district. If the substitute has been approved by another local board and comes with good recommendations, ask whether your board will extend the courtesy of accepting the prior board's approval so the substitute does not have to pay for another criminal background check.

- Ask the administration to add a listing seeking school nurse substitutes to any classified ad relating to employment in the district that runs in a newspaper or is posted on the district website.

C. Compromise:
- If substitute nurses cannot work the full day, have them work half days (and ask that pay be provided for the full day). Coordinate to have one work the morning and be relieved by another after lunch.

D. Make the substitute nurses' day as easy as possible:
- Do *not* leave extra work for them. Ask that they focus only on first aid.
- If health classes are scheduled, try to relieve them of this task as well as any nonnursing tasks such as attendance or hall duty.

E. Discourage your administration from calling a nursing agency to arrange for coverage:
- Nurses provided by an agency will probably not have formal school nurse training. There will be no means to evaluate performance, and student care can be compromised.
- The district might choose to hire an emergency nurse on a full-time basis to save the cost of benefits, leaving you out of a job.

F. Remember . . .
- Your contract is with the district, *not* with a particular school. It is within the rights of the employer to send you wherever they wish. This could include covering more than one school.
- If you must travel for an emergency or more frequently, do so without complaining. Put your concerns for student safety during your absence in writing, stressing the need for your presence in one location, *not* your inconvenience.
- Do not give up trying to recruit. If one suggestion does not work, try another.

TOPIC 2: NO LUNCH, NO PREP, NO PRIVACY, *AND* NO ONE CARES!

Fast Facts

School nurses, especially if they are new and not yet certified, frequently work through the day without stopping for breaks—lunch, coffee, bathroom, or preparation times.

(continued)

(continued)

Clinical Snapshot

Kim eagerly accepted a position in a local, urban middle school with an enrollment of just over 800 students. As there were no other applicants and her two predecessors left midyear, Kim was given emergency certification and began immediately. Kim's school has five children with diabetes, 12 with anaphylaxis, two with seizure disorders, and numerous asthmatic students as well as others with chronic diseases. Preparation time is inconceivable, nor does she *ever* have a duty-free lunch.

Frustrated, one day when she is unable to make a 10-minute private call to check on her ill son, Kim overcame the fear of losing her job and informed the principal that she needs uninterrupted time during the day. His response is, "I never get lunch either."

Suggested School Nurse Actions

A. Investigate the terms of your contract. Unless the school nurse's position is addressed separately, you have the same benefits as your teacher colleagues. This includes lunch and preparation periods.

B. Attempt to work with your principal and colleagues to develop a health office schedule. Perhaps the first hours of the morning and afternoon sessions could be designated as clinic times during which nonurgent care is rendered and you see any student sent to you. The remainder of the day would be for screenings, writing, and addressing immediate needs. The quietest time of the day, usually midmorning or late afternoon, could be lunch or prep time for you.

C. Speak, in confidence, with your union representative to alert him or her of the situation. This may raise broader concerns since the teachers bargained for these rights. If they are denied to you, the administration may expect others to do likewise.

D. Request additional help. Suggest the district hire a registered professional nurse to work on an hourly basis for even 1 or 2 hours a day. Emphasize that this nurse would also be someone comfortable covering in your absence and the cost would be minimal. Stress the safety factor in having adequate coverage for the school's medically fragile students. If this nurse is competent, encourage her or him to consider pursuing additional preparation to become a school nurse. Offer to help the nurse reach this goal.

TOPIC 3: HEALTHCARE AVAILABILITY

Fast Facts

The Centers for Disease Control and Prevention (CDC) reported that the percentage of children without health insurance was 5.1% in 2017 (CDC, 2017). This equated to approximately one child out of every 20 who did not have medical benefits.

Clinical Snapshot

School nurse Kim is competent and caring but was unaware that one student's dad had lost his job, leaving the family without health benefits. The student has a chronic disease that requires medical management and long-term drug therapy. Kim should be aware of this family's temporary needs and refer them to agencies for help in finding appropriate medical care.

School nurses know better than anyone the importance of access to comprehensive, affordable health coverage. Unfulfilled health and mental needs can result in developmentally delayed children who struggle socially and academically. We know poor children have worse access to healthcare and can start school behind others.

Medicaid and the Children's Defense Fund work to ensure that all children have coverage and timely access to care.

Today the number of uninsured children is at a historic low. Medicaid can be offered to some, based on the family income. Medicaid is the single largest health insurer for children. It provides coverage at no cost.

As of February 2018, the Children's Health Insurance Program (CHIP) has been authorized to continue through the year 2027.

Suggested School Nurse Actions

A. Familiarize yourself with the families of your students, especially those with extensive medical needs, unemployment issues, or a transient lifestyle.
B. Question parents about healthcare coverage.
C. Link parents with services and rights to which they are entitled under the law.

D. Seek to make available donations of cash or food gift cards for families in need, no questions asked.
E. Consider participating in community projects to help stock local food pantries.

TOPIC 4: SCHOOL-SPONSORED BEFORE- AND AFTER-CARE PROGRAMS, ACTIVITIES, AND CLASS TRIPS

Fast Facts

Today's school day is quite different than that of the past. With so many working and single-parent homes, a significant number of children begin their day hours before the first class and stay in the building well into the evening. Class field trips are commonly scheduled every year, and all students participate. Those with special needs must be cared for by a registered professional nurse before and after school and while attending class trips.

Clinical Snapshot

Kim had planned to stay late to finish up some paperwork. For 2 hours, as she tries to complete this work, she is repeatedly interrupted by students who are involved in after-school sports, others who are in the after-school program, and parents who want to visit when they come to pick up their child. Kim is tempted to take some of the charts home to work on but resists the impulse, knowing that student health records are legal documents that should not leave the school.

Programs That Extend the School Day

Most districts have some plan to meet the needs of single parents and those whose workday extends beyond the normal school hours. Programs are offered that enable students to begin their day before the first class and extend into the early evening. Know the particulars of those that are independently run and those that are sponsored by the school.

Many schools also offer sports or extracurricular activities outside of the school day. For the school nurse, this means that she or he is virtually never in the building without children or staff present. If no substitute nurse is available to go on a field trip to administer medication, the school nurse must go. This means the rest of the school is left with no coverage.

Suggested School Nurse Actions

A. Review the protocol of providers who coordinate before- or after-care programs or other school events. If the program is not school sponsored and the care provider does not offer nursing coverage, make sure parents are aware of this.

B. Speak with your principal, and have him or her stress to staff that you should not be depended on for care outside of school hours.

C. Check with your union leaders to clarify your responsibilities if you are in the building off hours.

D. Try not to get caught while you are sitting or standing behind your desk. When a parent or staff member approaches and you do not have time to speak, greet them at your door or in the hallway. You can then excuse yourself and walk away without appearing rude.

E. If students with medical needs are participating in after-school sports, try to have a coach trained as a delegate for epinephrine or glucagon use.

F. If you are working before or after school hours, close your door and hide! Let no one know you are working. If there is a *true* emergency, they will find you, and for this occasional instance, you will certainly not mind being interrupted.

School-Sponsored Trips

In most schools, children go on a yearly class trip. It would be hurtful and possibly illegal to exclude a student from these activities because of a special need or lack of money. If a child in that class needs medication or a specific treatment, a nurse must accompany the class on the trip. This presents a problem as a substitute nurse must be provided either to go on the trip or to cover the school so you can go.

Suggested School Nurse Actions

A. In planning class trips, check to see whether a parent of the child with medical needs can attend. Have the teacher plan well in advance so parents have ample time to arrange their schedules.

B. See Topic 1 regarding suggestions for obtaining substitute nurses.

C. Investigate the possibility of keeping a small amount of money available to cover the costs for students who cannot afford to go on trips (or any other pressing need you are aware of). The names of those who access this money must be kept in confidence. Seek funding from the parent–teacher association or any group willing to trust your judgment.

D. If a child requires the use of epinephrine due to food allergies, check to see if a trained delegate may be permitted to go on the field trip in lieu of a substitute registered nurse.

TOPIC 5: MEDICALLY FRAGILE STUDENTS NEEDING ONE-ON-ONE CARE

Fast Facts

Today we recognize that children with chronic diseases or conditions are part of the mainstream. Bear in mind that the Individuals With Disabilities Education Act (IDEA; Wrightslaw, 1990) states that all children are entitled to *a free and public education in the least restrictive environment*. Some of these children are considered *nursing dependent* or *medically fragile* and may be *technology dependent* as well (Washington State Model).

Clinical Snapshot

Kim is fortunate that there is a competent nurse assigned to her nursing-dependent students. However, when the nurse is absent or problems arise, Kim must be prepared to intervene. The overwhelming accommodations needed for these special children can compromise Kim's available time for the remaining students.

Suggested School Nurse Actions

A. Participate in making the assessment of needs and recommending the level of care that the student with medical needs receives—health aide, licensed practical nurse, or registered nurse.

B. Meet with the child, parents, and other child study team members to perform the evaluation properly *before* the child is placed in class. You do *not* need to be part of the discussion of who pays for this service.

C. At the first meeting, question who carries full responsibility for the child's care. If the caregiver is an aide or a licensed practical nurse, you, as the certified school nurse, may be in charge. Put your questions and responses in writing, or make sure the discussion is part of the minutes for the meeting.

D. Clarify who is to care for the child if the designated individual is absent. If you are expected to step in, request that your office be covered by a substitute nurse.

E. Get to know the child and his or her needs. Even if one-on-one care is provided, the child is still your student.

F. Get to know the one-on-one provider. Check to be sure proper care is rendered and someone is evaluating the caregiver.

TOPIC 6: PROFESSIONAL RESPONSIBILITIES

Fast Facts

Administrators are sometimes reluctant to include you in meetings that require you to be out of your office. Someone must cover your calls and office visits, and realistically, no one wants to do this.

Clinical Snapshot

The director of special services has requested Kim's presence at a child study team meeting to assess the level of care necessary for a medically fragile child who will be attending her school. In preparation for the meeting, school nurse Kim researches the child's condition, reads the medical records, visits the child at home, observes the student in the current school placement, and speaks with the parents in anticipation for the meeting.

Kim informs the principal that she will be out of her office for the designated meeting time, yet she is called by the secretary to return to her office twice—first for a child who wet his pants and next for a child who was tired.

Suggested School Nurse Actions

A. *Before* any meeting you plan to attend, clarify who is to determine if you should be pulled from the meeting. A busy secretary might not want her work interrupted or may feel it is not her job to care for sick children.

B. Come to a mutual agreement with the administrator and secretary about what is expected in your absence and what constitutes an emergency.
C. Clarify who is in charge. If the director of special services or any administrator requires your participation in a meeting, the secretary should not be overriding the director's decision by summoning you out of the meeting for a nonemergency.
D. When discussing your professional performance with the administration, stress that the priorities of your tasks should be to *do what no other staff member can do*, not what the other staff member chooses *not to do*.
E. Do not accept the rationale that there is no one else who is available to help. In many cases, insisting on having a nurse to handle a situation is the path of least resistance. Rather than confronting the other staff member, administrators may continue to let nonnursing tasks fall on you because you will get the job done. However, you cannot be in two places at the same time, have numerous bosses, or remain excluded from participating in educational or medical planning that requires your input or for which only you are qualified.
F. Review your contract to see what rights the other teachers and staff members are given. If they are entitled to duty-free lunch and prep periods, you should be, too.
G. Accept that there may be times when your constant presence in the building will be necessary for the well-being of certain students. This is the nature of the beast. Investigate additional compensation, other local nurses who could cover, or a rotating nurse to cover all nurse lunches in the district.

TOPIC 7: UNLICENSED OR NONCERTIFIED PERSONNEL IN THE HEALTH OFFICE

Fast Facts

Ideally, every school should have *at least* one nurse who is certified in the specialty of school nursing.

Clinical Snapshot

Today's school health office is a busy place. When the enrollment is large or student needs are complex, health aides or health assistants may be necessary. These registered nurses provide needed help to the school nurse and are most welcome.

The problem arises when a district, often in an attempt to save money, permits a nurse who has had no preparation or experience as a school nurse to work independently. Frequently, the certified school nurse must serve as the supervisor for a noncertified nurse working in another building. The certified nurse may be legally responsible for the noncertified nurse's job performance.

Suggested School Nurse Actions

A. As positions arise within your district, encourage your administration to hire only properly credentialed nurses. When it comes to the health and safety of children, money should not be an issue.

B. All personnel must have a clearly written job description that does *not* conflict with the role of the certified school nurse. Check with your administration and union officials to make sure there is no confusion before a conflict arises.

C. If the district is unionized, the school nurse should be included in the contract. That means he or she pays dues as do the teachers and is entitled to be placed on salary guide and receive the same rights and benefits.

D. Secretaries or administrative assistants are a valuable help to the school nurse. They can handle phone calls, order supplies, and perform clerical tasks while working within their job description. They should *not* be involved in assessing students, conferencing with staff or parents, attending meetings on behalf of the school nurse, charting, or giving medications.

TOPIC 8: SCHOOL NURSE SUPERVISION AND EVALUATION; STUDENT GROWTH OBJECTIVES

Fast Facts

All schools have some type of evaluation process for professional staff. Unfortunately, school nurses are seldom evaluated by an administrator who truly understands what we do. Some districts are now using nationally recognized programs that provide a generic outline of items to be considered in evaluation.

(*continued*)

(continued)

Clinical Snapshot

Kim has been a school nurse for more than 20 years. She has had nothing but glowing evaluations from every administrator. However, no one has ever offered her constructive suggestions to better her practice.

Student growth objectives (SGOs) are the latest initiative introduced in some states to assess and improve student instruction. As a school nurse, you are considered a support specialist and may be obligated to partake in the requirements.

Suggested School Nurse Actions

A. Investigate the evaluation tool your district is using. If this tool is comprehensive, valid, and reflects what you do, accept it.
B. If you have questions on the effectiveness of the evaluation tool, raise your concerns *before* you are evaluated. Once the evaluation is completed, you will have little chance to have it altered.
C. Consider obtaining administrative or supervisory certification yourself so that you can evaluate other school nurses. It would be more beneficial if our evaluations contained constructive suggestions for improvement from a knowledgeable source.
D. If you have been told you must write SGOs, the objectives you have previously identified for your own practice might serve as a guide. You might wish to spend less time on nonnursing tasks or have all your individualized healthcare plans (IHPs) completed by a certain date. You can also work with colleagues to formulate district-wide objectives.
E. Find your own school nurse role model to guide you to a better nursing practice. We all can improve in some way.

TOPIC 9: PEDICULOSIS

Fast Facts

The American Association of Pediatrics (AAP) and the National Association of School Nurses (NASN) agree that no-nit policies in schools should be *discontinued* (NASN, 2016).

(continued)

(*continued*)

Clinical Snapshot

School nurse Kim spends the entire month of September looking through children's heads for lice. The nurse who preceded her told her this was expected.

Head lice are probably responsible for more wasted school nurse hours than any other issue. Teachers panic, administrators do not know what to do, and parents will drive you insane when a child is identified with pediculosis. School nurses know that lice cause no threat to health, lice are nothing more than a nuisance, and, in terms of protecting students from illness, our time would be better spent doing a daily temperature check on every student.

Children found to have head lice should remain in class but be discouraged from close direct head contact with others. The educational process should not be disrupted (NASN, 2016).

Suggested School Nurse Actions

A. Research your school policy. If you have a no-nit policy, seek to change it *before* there are reported cases to deal with. Education is the key here, and it cannot be provided effectively in the middle of an outbreak. Educate before the problem manifests, when parents, staff, and administration are more receptive. Unlike the body and pubic louse, the head louse *prefers* a clean host because it can easily grasp the hair follicle. The body louse lives in the seams of dirty clothing, and the pubic louse is an sexually transmitted infection. These two are associated with uncleanliness, *not* the head louse.

B. If a case is reported, check that student and his or her siblings. If several cases are seen in the same class, check the entire class. Mass schoolwide screenings are *not* necessary. Check students at the end of the school day. This way if a case is detected, the child will be going home shortly, and it will not be necessary to embarrass him or her by summoning a parent from work for an early dismissal. Notify the parent by phone. Check the student the following day to be sure he or she has been treated, and allow the child to return. Refer parents to a physician for information about the best treatment product, as you would with any other disease.

C. Send a notice home in September regarding all communicable diseases (streptococcal infections, viruses, impetigo, coxsackie, conjunctivitis, lice, etc.). List the symptoms to watch for, and explain that these diseases are commonly seen in school-age children. For the parents who *insist* that a notice about communicable diseases be sent home, *you have already done it!* This notice early in the school year is also a good time to remind parents to keep the ill children at home, send a note upon return, and clarify when a physician's clearance is required for return to school.

D. With administrative approval, consider sending a separate notice home only if you have numerous cases of lice, conjunctivitis, or any other disease.

E. Refuse to disclose the names of infected children. Suggest that parents notify the playmates of affected children.

TOPIC 10: PRIORITIZING TASKS

Fast Facts

Always put the needs of the students first. Reports, charting, administrative demands, meetings, phone calls, and so on can all wait.

Clinical Snapshot

Kim has finished her required school nurse coursework and has landed her long-anticipated job. Now she is overwhelmed by the numerous tasks before her. She takes a deep breath, relaxes, and starts to prioritize what must be done immediately and what can be put temporarily on the back burner.

Suggested School Nurse Actions

A. **Contact Information**

- Make sure every adult and child in the building has a current emergency card that is completed, signed, and available in your office.

Students

- Do not discard the previous year's cards; you may need to refer to them for additional phone contacts. Include a section that parents can use for updating any recent health concerns involving their child.

Faculty and Staff

- Include a few blank lines that the teacher can initial for the next year if there are no changes or use for updating any new issues.

B. Children With Special Needs

Identify

- Review health data for each child: Physical exams, former school records, medications, restrictions, treatments, and so on.
- Place the information in individual folders.
- Ask the previous school nurse, secretary, and teachers to share any health information with you.
- Contact each parent or guardian to request updated information.
- Obtain written permission to share information with those who have a need to know.

Develop List

- Write a confidential list, for your use only, of all children with special needs.
- Meet with every child's teacher, and share what and with whom you have been given permission to share.
- Do not distribute copies of the list.

Recordkeeping

- Write IHPs and emergency care plans (ECPs) for those in need.
- Use reference books or software programs to develop a standard format for these plans.
- Check to see if your colleagues have IHPs they would be willing to share, and adapt them for your students. If there are no changes from the previous year, you and the child's parents can just sign off on the prior year's plan for the upcoming year.

C. Medications

Identify

- Check to be sure you have medications for all children who *need* to be dosed during the school day. You will want to have the medication, along with the permission slips from the parent and physician, on hand before the child starts school. Check expiration dates, physician's orders, and parental consents.

Develop List

- Write down the names of those children needing daily medications and those with prn orders.
- Create a binder or computer-generated portfolio with separate charting sheets for each child.

Recordkeeping

- Chart immediately after each dose is given.

Tips

- Give medication only to the child whose name is indicated on the container—no sharing.
- Count controlled medications with the adult who brings them in.
- Insist that all medications be provided in their original containers.
- Keep all medications locked, except those needed for emergency administration.
- Have a stock nebulizer, tubing, and epinephrine available.
- Place epinephrine and glucagon in a safe, secure, unlocked location.
- Check delegates training form for each child.
- Attach each child's ECP and contact information with his or her medication.

D. Immunizations

Identify

- Make an outline of all the state-required immunizations, and post it on your desk for immediate reference.
- Get an updated list of the entire school population according to class or grade.
- Have a health folder for every student, including those placed out of district.
- Review all immunization dates, comparing the time sequence with the birth date.

Develop List

- Prepare a form that you can use as a checklist to ensure that all required health documents and immunizations have been received. Include the student's name, birth date, date of last physical exam, and so on.
- Send the form out to parents of children whose records are incomplete, indicating what is needed, and give a deadline for submission.
- Keep a list of those students who are deficient in immunizations.
- If the response from parents is not timely, send second notice, and copy your administrator.
- If the parents still do not respond, ask your administrator to intervene and threaten exclusion.

Recordkeeping

- For those whose records appear complete, place information in the child's folder to be filled in at a later date.

E. Standing Orders

Identify

- Identify the procedures you and the school physician feel are appropriate for delivering healthcare to students. If you do not have standing orders, ask colleagues in neighboring districts if they will share theirs, and adapt them for your district.

Develop List

- Review the standing orders carefully, and make changes as needed. You may only order supplies included in your standing orders.

Recordkeeping

- Review and have the orders signed annually by the school physician. This is best done in June in preparation for the following school year.

Appendix C, Month-by-Month Calendar of Tasks, will give you further insight into what must be done immediately.

References

Centers for Disease Control and Prevention. (2017). *Health Insurance Coverage*. Retrieved from https://www.cdc.gov/nchs/fastats/health-insurance.htm

National Association of School Nurses. (2016). *Head lice management in the school setting. Position statement 2004*. Retrieved from https://www.nasn.org/advocacy/...practicedocuments/position-statements/ps-head-lice

Wrightslaw. (1990). *IDEA: Least restrictive environment (LRE) and free appropriate public education free appropriate public education (FAPE)*. Retrieved from https://www.wrightslaw.com/advoc/articles/idea.lre.fape.htm

Appendix A
Healthy People 2020 Topics

A

Access to Health Services
Adolescent Health (*New*)
Arthritis, Osteoporosis, and Chronic Back Conditions

B

Blood Disorders and Blood Safety (*New*)

C

Cancer
Chronic Kidney Disease

D

Dementias, Including Alzheimer's Disease (*New*)
Diabetes
Disability and Health

E

Early and Middle Childhood (*New*)
Educational and Community-Based Programs
Environmental Health

F

Family Planning
Food Safety

G

Genomics (*New*)
Global Health (*New*)

H

Health Communication and Health Information Technology
Healthcare-Associated Infections (*New*)
Health-Related Quality of Life and Well-Being (*New*)
Hearing and Other Sensory or Communication Disorders
Heart Disease and Stroke
HIV

I

Immunization and Infectious Diseases
Injury and Violence Prevention

L

Lesbian, Gay, Bisexual, and Transgender Health (*New*)

M

Maternal, Infant, and Child Health
Medical Product Safety
Mental Health and Mental Disorders

N

Nutrition and Weight Status

O

Occupational Safety and Health
Older Adults (*New*)
Oral Health

P

Physical Activity
Preparedness (*New*)
Public Health Infrastructure

R

Respiratory Diseases

S

Sexually Transmitted Diseases
Sleep Health (*New*)
Social Determinants of Health (*New*)
Substance Abuse

T

Tobacco Use

V

Vision

Source: Adapted from *Healthy People 2020*. (n.d.). *Topics and Objectives—Objectives A–Z*. U.S. Department of Health and Human Services. Retrieved from www.healthypeople.gov/2020/topicsobjectives2020/.

Appendix B
Health Office Setup

FIRST-AID SUPPLIES

- Bandages
- Ice packs
- Arm and leg splints
- Soap and other antiseptics
- Paper towels
- Eyewash setup

EQUIPMENT

- Privacy screen
- File cabinet
- Desk
- Swivel chair
- Cot with paper roll
- Double-lock medicine cabinet
- Dedicated phone line
- Refrigerator large enough for medications and ice packs
- Several chairs
- Air conditioner
- Computer

ASSESSMENT TOOLS

- Several types of thermometers
- Blood pressure machine with adult and pediatric cuffs

- Stethoscope
- Audiometer
- Vision testing equipment
- Scoliometer
- Height, growth, and basal metabolic index (BMI) charts
- Scale
- Pulse oximeter

BATHROOM

- Window or exhaust system
- Doorway wide enough to permit wheelchair access
- Sink with eyewash station

Appendix C
Month-by-Month Calendar of Tasks

*AUGUST

1. Unpack supplies. Clean and prepare the office for the first day of school.
2. Review information on incoming students. Set up charts.
3. Send written notices or make phone calls if deficiencies are found in examination or immunization records.
4. Note students with specific medical needs.
5. Formulate a student-alert list for your own reference. Do not disseminate it to entire staff.
6. Check standing orders. Update as needed.
7. Review individualized healthcare plans and emergency health plans from the previous year. Write plans for new students.
8. Check students who receive medication in school; review physician orders, parental consents, asthma action plans, and so on.
9. Contact parents who have children with severe allergies, asthma, or seizure disorders. Get medications and paperwork before students enter school.
10. Check expiration dates on all medications.
11. Check locks on medication and supply cabinets.
12. Prepare plans for substitute nurses.
13. Formulate goals for the new school year.

*Look into getting paid for these noncontractual hours. If other members of the child study team are compensated, you may be entitled also.

SEPTEMBER

1. Have students' folders arranged by class or grade level.
2. Make sure all students have had state-required immunizations. File an immunization status report if it is required by your state.
3. Meet individually with teachers to review students' health needs.
4. Introduce yourself to new students, teachers, and parents.
5. Distribute, collect, and review emergency information for students and staff.
6. Conduct a staff in-service education program covering the Heimlich maneuver, automated external defibrillator (AED), glucagon, and epinephrine auto-injector. Distribute universal precaution supplies.
7. Check on staff certifications for cardiopulmonary resuscitation and AED use. Arrange renewals as needed.
8. Organize epinephrine auto-injector and glucagon delegates, and have consent forms signed. Do training.
9. Begin tuberculosis testing.
10. Review team assignments: crisis, 504, intervention and referral, child study.
11. Review previous year's goals, student growth outcomes, and professional improvement plans. Formulate new ones.
12. Check health folders. Review each class list, making sure you have a folder for every child.

OCTOBER

1. Begin screenings: height and weight.
2. Start blood pressure screenings.

NOVEMBER

1. Review and update individual healthcare and emergency plans.
2. Continue screenings: Vision and hearing.

DECEMBER

1. Continue screenings: Vision and hearing.

JANUARY

1. Continue screenings: Vision and hearing.
2. Review documentation for all students: Check immunizations, referrals, deficiencies, care plans, medications, and so on.

FEBRUARY

1. Continue screenings: Dental and blood pressure.
2. Check outdoor playground equipment for damage from winter months.

MARCH

1. Continue screenings: Basal metabolic index (BMI).
2. Conduct kindergarten registration. Review incoming students' records.

APRIL

1. Continue screenings: Scoliosis.
2. Review goals for the school year. Begin to formulate new goals for the upcoming year.

MAY

1. Begin charting screening results. Follow up on all outstanding referrals.
2. Review and update standing orders.
3. Order supplies for the new school year.
4. Make teacher recommendations for students with special needs.

JUNE

1. Prepare an annual report.
2. Close out documentation, and transfer information to sending schools.

3. Notify parents to obtain medications. Send medication permission slips out for the coming school year. Return unused medications to parents.
4. Have standing orders signed by the school physician to cover the upcoming school year.
5. Dispose of medical waste (e.g., sharps) according to district policy.
6. Review records of incoming students, inform parents of deficiencies, and set up folders.
7. Transfer records, and give verbal reports on outgoing students to receiving nurses.
8. Do a supply inventory. Order supplies as needed.
9. Prepare an annual report.
10. Send notices for students requiring physical examinations in September.
11. Send equipment out for calibration.

Appendix D
National Health Observances

Month	Primary Topics	Alternate Topics
January	Healthy weight	Blood donation Drug and alcohol awareness
February	Dental health	Burn awareness Date violence Heart health
March	Nutrition	Red Cross Poison prevention Diabetes awareness Violence prevention
April	Autism	Earth Day Alcohol awareness Child abuse prevention Sexual assault prevention World health Every Kid Healthy Air quality
May	Asthma	Skin cancer Food allergy Mental health Hand hygiene Walk and bike to school Safe swimming
June	Headache	Home safety Fireworks safety Safety
July	Eye injury	Fireworks safety
August	Immunizations	Medic alert

(continued)

(*continued*)

Month	Primary Topics	Alternate Topics
September	Injury prevention	Alcohol and drugs Fruits and vegetables Obesity awareness Food safety Pediculosis prevention Traumatic brain injury Suicide prevention School backpack Family fitness
October	Heart health	Fire prevention Walk to school Bully prevention Depression screening
November	Smoking cessation	Diabetes
December	Handwashing	Safe toys World AIDS

Source: Adapted from National Health Information Center. (2011). *National health observances*. Washington, DC: Office of Disease Prevention and Health Promotion, U.S. Department of Health and Human Services. Retrieved from http://healthfinder.gov; National Wellness Institute. (2011). *Health observances*. Retrieved from NationalWellness.org; and Wellness Council of America. (2018). *National Health Observances & Awareness Months*. Retrieved from https://www.welcoa.org/health-observances/.

Glossary

504 accommodation plan An accommodation plan for children who have been identified with learning and other types of disabilities under the Rehabilitation Act of 1973–Section 504

Americans With Disability Act (ADA) The 1990 law that prohibits discrimination against people with disabilities in all areas of public life—jobs, school, transportation, and places open to the public

Body mass index (BMI) A measure of body fat based on a calculation that involves height and weight

Child Abuse Prevention and Treatment Act (CAPTA) The 1974 law that provides federal funding to states in support of child abuse prevention, assessment, prosecution, and treatment activities

Child protective services agency The name given to a government agency in many states that responds to reports of child abuse

Child study team A group of professionals typically employed by a board of education to provide parents and teachers with a variety of learning-related services for the child with special needs

Coordinated school health program A systematic approach to improving the health and well-being of all students so they can fully participate and be successful in school

Culture Behaviors and beliefs characteristic of a particular social, ethnic, or age group

Cultural competency The ability to interact effectively with people of different cultures and socioeconomic backgrounds

Cultural diversity The coexistence of different ethnic, gender, racial, and socioeconomic groups within one social unit

Cultural sensitivity Consciousness and understanding of the morals, standards, and principles of a specific culture, society, ethnic group, or race, joined by a motivation to acclimate one's actions with such

Curriculum content standards The health knowledge and skills students should know and be able to perform at different educational levels

Emergency care plan (ECP) A plan written for a student who could present a classroom emergency due to a medical condition; it indicates what to do if the emergency happens, the medication to give, and whom to call and should also include a picture of the student

Health literacy Competence in critical thinking and problem-solving leading to responsible and productive behaviors

***Healthy People* initiative** The comprehensive, nationwide health-promotion and disease-prevention agenda, revised every 10 years to meet specific health objectives

Individualized education plan (IEP) A document mandated by the Individuals With Disabilities Education Act (IDEA) that defines individual goals for a child with a disability

Individualized healthcare plan (IHP) A proposed sequence of actions developed by the school nurse using the nursing process to meet the health needs of a student

Individuals With Disabilities Education Act (IDEA) The 1990 federal special-education law that ensures that all schools serve the educational needs of students with disabilities

Licensed practical nurse (LPN) A nurse who cares for the sick, injured, or disabled under the supervision of a registered nurse or physician; in California and Texas, known as a *licensed vocational nurse*

Morbid obesity The state of being more than 100 pounds above one's ideal body weight; indicated by a BMI over 40

Obese A medical condition in which excess weight negatively affects one's health and life expectancy; indicated by a BMI over 30

Registered professional nurse A nurse who has graduated from a nursing program at a college or university and has passed a national licensing exam

Further Reading

Advameg. (2010). *Mainstreaming*. Retrieved from http://www.faqs.org/health/topics/2/Mainstreaming.html

American Nurses Association. (1998). *Scope and standards of professional school nurse practice*. Silver Spring, MD: Author.

American Academy of Pediatrics. (2008). Disaster planning for schools. *Pediatrics, 122*(4), 895–901. doi:10.1542/peds.2008-2170

American Nurses Association & National Council of State Boards of Nursing. (2013). *Principles for delegation by registered nurses to unlicensed assistive personnel*. Retrieved from https://www.ncsbn.org/Delegation_joint_statement_NCSBN-ANA.pdf

American Nurses Association & National Council of State Boards of Nursing. (n.d.) *Joint statement on delegation*. Retrieved from www.ncsbn.org/Delegation_joint_statement_NCSBN-ANA.pdf

Autism Speaks. (2018). *What is autism?* Retrieved from https://www.autismspeaks.org/what-autism

Berg, F. (2004). *Underage and overweight: America's childhood obesity crisis: What every family needs to know* (pp. 3–33). Long Island City, NY: Hatherleigh Press.

Bosch, C. (1997). *Schools under siege: Issues in focus* (pp. 5–17, 77–91). Springfield, NJ: Enslow.

Bowman, R. (1994). *Cultural diversity and academic achievement*. Retrieved from http://www.ncrel.org/sdrs/areas/issues/educators/leadrshp/le0bow.htm

Centers for Disease Control and Prevention. (2008). *Childhood obesity facts*. Retrieved from https://www.cdc.gov//obesity/data/childhood.html

Centers for Disease Control and Prevention. (2009). *Health insurance coverage: Early release of estimates for the national health interview survey, 200d*. Retrieved from https://www.cdc.gov/nchs/data/nhis/earlyrelease/Insur201808.pdf

Centers for Disease Control and Prevention. (2010). *Morbidity and mortality weekly report* (June 4, 2010). Retrieved from http://www.cdc.gov/mmwr/pdf/ss/ss5905.pdf

Centers for Disease Control and Prevention. (2013a). *National health education standards*. Retrieved from https://www.cdc.gov/healthyschools/sher/standards/index.htm

Centers for Disease Control and Prevention. (2019). *Birth-18 years immunization schedule*. Retrieved from https://www.cdc.gov/vaccines/schedules/hcp/imz/child-adolescent.html

Centers for Disease Control and Prevention. (n.d.-a). *Body mass index age–percentile charts for boys and girls*. Retrieved online from http://www.cdc.gov/healthyweight/assessing/bmi/childrens_bmi/about_childrens_bmi.html

Centers for Disease Control and Prevention. (n.d.-b). *Drug overdose deaths*. Retrieved from https://www.cdc.gov/drugoverdose/data/statedeaths.html

Centers for Disease Control and Prevention. (n.d.-c). *Fact Sheet: Physical school environment*. Retrieved from https://www.cdc.gov/HealthyYouth/SHPPS/2006/factsheets/pdf/FS_PhysicalSchoolEnvironment_SHPPS2006.pdf

Centers for Disease Control and Prevention. (n.d.-d). *Head lice information for schools*. Retrieved from https://www.cdc.gov/parasites/lice/head/schools.html

Centers for Disease Control and Prevention. (n.d.-e). *Mental health*. Retrieved from https://www.cdc.gov/childrensmentalhealth/data.html

Centers for Disease Control and Prevention. (n.d.-f). *School connectedness | Protective factors | Adolescent and school health*. Retrieved from https://www.cdc.gov/healthyyouth/protective/school_connectedness.htm

Centers for Disease Control and Prevention. (n.d.-g). *Signs and symptoms of autism spectrum disorders*. Retrieved from https://www.cdc.gov/ncbddd/autism/signs.html

Centers for Disease Control and Prevention. (n.d.-h). *Youth risk behavior surveillance system*. Retrieved from https://www.cdc.gov/healthyyouth/data/yrbs/index.htm

Davidson, T. (2003). *School conflict* (pp. 34–35). New York, NY: Scholastic.

Eaton, D. K., Kann, L., Kinchen, S., Shanklin, S., Ross, J., Hawkins, J., . . . Wechsler, H. (2010, June 4). Youth risk behavior surveillance—United States, 2009. *Morbidity and Mortality Weekly Report*. Retrieved from http://cdc.gov/mmwr/preview/mmwrhtml/ss5905a1.htm

Faracone, S. (2003). *Straight talk about your child's mental health: What to do when something seems wrong*. New York, NY: Guilford Press.

Forbes. (n.d.). *14 signs of an adaptable person*. Retrieved from https://www.forbes.com/sites/jeffboss/2015/09/03/14-signs-of-an-adaptable-person/

Good Choices Good Life. (n.d.). *How to respect yourself and others*. Retrieved from http://www.goodchoicesgoodlife.org/choices-for-young-people/r-e-s-p-e-c-t/

Grant, J. A. (2015, September 21). *Why curiosity in business is a winning attribute*. Retrieved from https://janeadsheadgrant.com/index.php/2015/09/21/why-curiosity-in-business-is-a-winning-attribute/

Grapes, B. J. (Ed.). (2001). *Child abuse: Contemporary issues companion*. San Diego, CA: Greenhaven Press.

Great Schools. (n.d.). *School attendance: Issues to consider*. Retrieved from http://www.greatschools.org/parenting/behavior-discipline/school-attendance-issues.gs/com

Healthy People 2010. (n.d.-a). Retrieved from http://www.healthypeople.gov/2020/default.aspx

Healthy People 2010. (n.d.-b). *Final review.* Retrieved from https://www.cdc.gov/nchs/healthy_people/hp2010/hp2010_final_review.htm

Healthy People 2020. (n.d.-c). *Topics and objectives—Objectives A-Z.* Retrieved from www.healthypeople.gov/2020/topicsobjectives2020/

Healthy People 2030. Office of Disease Prevention and Health Promotion *Healthy People 2030.* (n.d.). Retrieved from healthypeople.gov

HHS.gov. (n.d.). *Cultural competence.* Retrieved from https://www.hhs.gov/ash/oah/resources-and-training/tpp-and-paf-resources/cultural-competence/index.html

Kutscher, M. L. (2005). *Kids in the syndrome mix.* Philadelphia, PA: Jessica Kingsley.

LawHelp. (n.d.). *The differences between federal, state, and local laws.* Retrieved from https://www.lawhelp.org/resource/the-differences-between-federal-state-and-loc

Lifehack. (n.d.). *4 reasons why curiosity is important and how to develop it.* Retrieved from https://www.lifehack.org/articles/productivity/4-reasons-why-curiosity-is-important-and-how-to-develop-it.html

Lynch, E. W., & Hanson, M. J. (1992). *Developing cross-cultural competence* (pp. 35–59). Baltimore, MD: Paul H. Brookes.

Mainstreaming. (2009). Retrieved September from http://www.faqs.org/health/topics/2/Mainstreaming.html

Marin, P., & Brown, B. (2008). *The school environment and adolescent well-being: Beyond academics. Child trends research brief* (p. 26). San Francisco, CA: National Adolescent and Young Adult Health Information Center.

Maslow, A. H. (1943). A theory of human motivation. *Psychology Review, 50*(4), 370–396. doi:10.1037/h0054346

McLeod, S. A. (2007). *Maslow's hierarchy of needs.* Retrieved from http://www.simplepsychology.org/maslow.html

Mindbodygreen. (n.d.). *How to stay present even when you feel like you can't.* Retrieved from https://www.mindbodygreen.com/0-8795/how-to-stay-present-evenwhen-you-feel-like-you-cant.html

National Association of School Nurses. (2002). *The use of telehealth technology in the practice of school nursing. Position statement.* Silver Spring, MD: Author.

National Association of School Nurses. (2004). *School health records. Issue brief.* Silver Spring, MD: Author.

National Association of School Nurses. (2005). *Environmental impact concerns in the school setting. Position statement.* Silver Spring, MD: Author.

National Association of School Nurses. (2006). *Disaster preparedness: School nurse role.* Retrieved from http://www.nasn.org/Default.aspx?tabid=221

National Association of School Nurses. (2011). *Pediculosis management in the school setting. Position statement* (rev. ed.). Silver Spring, MD: Author.

National Association of School Nurses. (2014). *Our history. Position statement.* Silver Spring, MD: Author.

National Association of School Nurses, Educational Recommendations. (2012, January). *Position statement.* Retrieved from https://www.nasn.org/nasn/advocacy/professional-practice-documents/position-statements

National Board for Certification of School Nurses. (2014). *Certification examination for school nurses handbook*. New York: Author. Retrieved from www.nbcsn.org

National Board of Certified School Nurses, National School Nurse Certification. (n.d.). Retrieved from nbcsn.org/examination

National Center for Educational Statistics. (2014). *The condition of education, indicator 13, children and youth with disabilities*. Retrieved February from http://nces.ed.gov/pubs2014/2014083.pdf

National Health Information Center. (2011). *National health observances*. Washington, DC: Office of Disease Prevention and Health Promotion, U.S. Department of Health and Human Services. Retrieved from http://healthfinder.gov

National Wellness Institute. (2011). *Health observances*. Retrieved from NationalWellness.org

Newton, J., Adams, R., & Marcontel, M. (1997). *The new school health handbook: A ready reference for school nurses and educators* (3rd ed., pp. 15–16, 353–364, 371–375). Paramus, NJ: Prentice-Hall.

Offit, P. A. (2008). *Autism's false prophets*. New York, NY: Columbia University Press.

Parent Center Hub. (n.d.). Retrieved from https://www.parentcenterhub.org/wp-content/uploads/repo_items/gr3.pdf

Pigott, D. C., & Kazzi, Z. N. (2007). Biological agents of concern. In T. G. Veneema (Ed.), *Disaster nursing and emergency preparedness for chemical, biological, and radiological terrorism and other hazards* (p. 404). New York: Springer Publishing Company.

PsychCentral. (n.d.). The importance of developing curiosity. Retrieved from https://psychcentral.com/blog/the-importance-of-developing-curiosity

Psychology Today. (n.d.). *Autism*. Retrieved from https://www.psychologytoday.com/us/basics/autism

Russo, C. (Ed.). (2006). *Key legal issues for schools*. Lanham, MA: Rowman and Littlefield Education.

Sacks, A. (2001). *Special education: A reference handbook* (pp. 43–58). Santa Barbara, CA: ABC-CLIO.

Saisan, J., Smith, M., & Segal, J. (2009). *Child abuse and neglect: Recognizing and preventing child abuse*. Retrieved from http://helpguide.org/mental/child_abuse_physical_emotional_sexual_neglect.htm

Saugus.net. (1998). *Glossary of computer terms*. Retrieved from https://www.saugus.net/Computer/Terms/

Schantz, S. (2010). What's new in the world of childhood obesity? *NASN School Nurse, 25*(6), 288–292.

Schmidt, H. (2016). Chronic disease prevention and health promotion. In *Public health ethics: Cases spanning the globe*. Retrieved from https://www.ncbi.nlm.nih.gov/books/NBK435779/

Schoessler, S. (2002, May 18). *Bits and bytes: Technology for the school health office*. Paper presented at Bergen County School Nurses Association, Woodridge, NJ.

Selekman, J. (Ed.). (2013). *School nursing: A comprehensive text* (2nd ed., p. 31), Philadelphia, PA: F. A. Davis.

Simons, J. A., Irwin, D. B., & Drinnien, B. A. (1987). Maslow's hierarchy of needs. In *Psychology: The search for understanding*. New York, NY: West Publishing.

Success. (2016, November 3). *Do you have adaptability?* Retrieved from www.success.com/article/do-you-have-adaptability

Summerfield, L. M. (1995, October). National standards for school health education. Why have health instruction in the schools? ERIC Digest Series. ED387483. Retrieved from https://eric.ed.gov/?id=ED387483

Trickett, P. K., & Schellenbach, C. J. (1998). *Violence against children in the family and community*. Washington, DC: American Psychological Association.

U.S. Department of Health and Human Services. (1997). *A research based guide for parents, educators and community leaders* (2nd ed.). Retrieved from http://www.healthypeople.gov

U.S. Department of Health and Human Services. (n.d.-a). *2009 national youth risk behavior surveillance report*. Retrieved from http://www.cdc.gov/mmwr/pdf/ss/ss5905.pdf

U.S. Department of Health and Human Services. (n.d.-b). *The Affordable Care Act*. Retrieved from http://www.hhs.gov/healthcare/rights/

U.S. Secret Service and U.S. Department of Education. (2002). *Threat assessment in school: A guide to managing threatening situations and to creating safe school climates*. Washington, DC: Author.

Veenema, T. G., Benitez, J., & Benware, S. (2007). Chemical agents of concern. In T. G. Veneema (Ed.), *Disaster nursing and emergency preparedness for chemical, biological, and radiological terrorism and other hazards* (p. 484). New York, NY: Springer Publishing Company.

Volokh, A., & Snell, L. (1998). *Strategies to keep schools safe*. Retrieved from https://reason.org/policy-study/strategies-to-keep-schools-saf/

Washington State Office of Superintendent of Public Instruction. (2000). *Levels of nursing care for student diseases and conditions: Severity coding. Staff model for the delivery of school health services* (pp. 8–24). Author.

Wellness Council of America. (2011). *Health observances*. Retrieved from https://www.welcoa.org/health-observances/

Wellness Council of America. (2018). *National Health Observances & Awareness Months*. Retrieved from https://www.welcoa.org/health-observances/

WikiJob. (n.d.). *Top 10 interpersonal skills: What they are, why they're important*. Retrieved from https://www.wikijob.co.uk/content/interview-advice/competencies/interpersonal-skills

Wolfe, D., & Mash, E. (Eds.). (2006). *Behavioral and emotional disorders in adolescents: Nature, assessment and treatment* (pp. 2–34, 535–540). New York, NY: Guilford Publications.

World Health Organization. (n.d.). *Health Education*. Retrieved from www.who.int/topics/health_education/en/

Zaiger, D. (2000). *School nursing practice: An orientation manual* (2nd ed.). Castle Rock, CO: National Association of School Nurses.

Index

FAST FACTS FOR YOUR NURSING CAREER

Choose from Over 45 Titles!

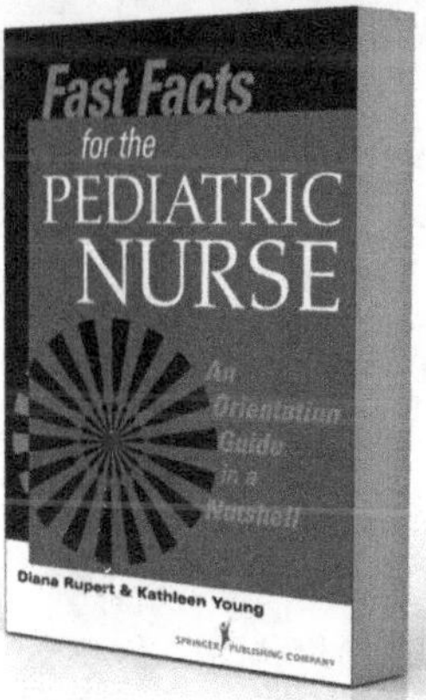

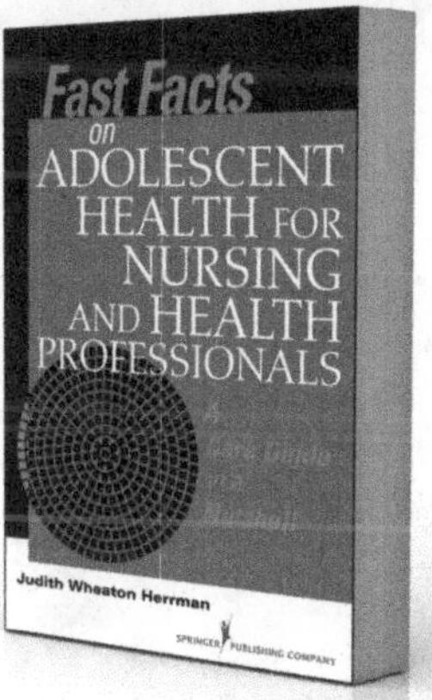

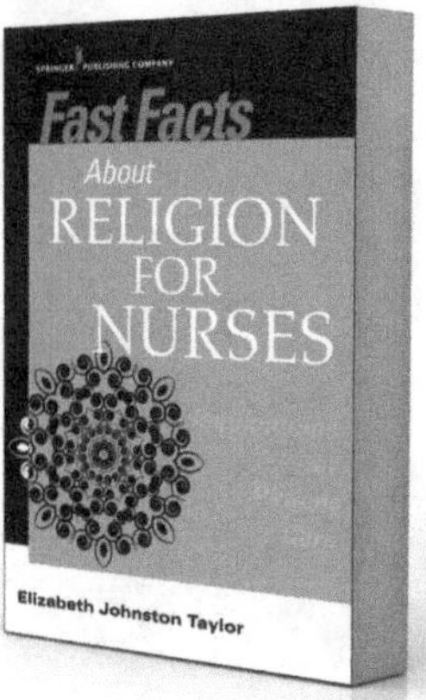

These must-have reference books are packed with timely, useful, and accessible information presented in a clear, precise format. Pocket-sized and affordable, the series provides quick access to information you need to know and use daily.

springerpub.com/FastFacts

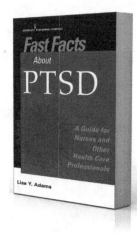

Printed in the United States
By Bookmasters